PSYCHIATRIC CASE FORMULATIONS

PSYCHIATRIC CASE FORMULATIONS

Len Sperry, M.D., Ph.D.

*Associate Professor of Psychiatry,
Medical College of Wisconsin, Milwaukee, Wisconsin*

Jon E. Gudeman, M.D.

*Professor and Co-Chairman, Department of Psychiatry,
Medical College of Wisconsin, Milwaukee, Wisconsin*

Barry Blackwell, M.D.

*Professor and Chairman, Department of Psychiatry,
University of Wisconsin Medical School, Milwaukee Clinical Campus,
Milwaukee, Wisconsin*

Larry R. Faulkner, M.D.

*Professor and Chairman,
Department of Neuropsychiatry and Behavioral Science,
University of South Carolina Medical School,
Columbia, South Carolina*

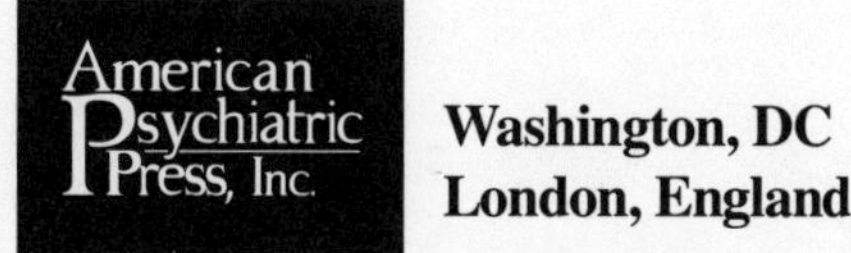

Washington, DC
London, England

Note: The authors have worked to ensure that all information in this book concerning drug dosages, schedules, and routes of administration is accurate as of the time of publication and consistent with standards set by the U.S. Food and Drug Administration and the general medical community. As medical research and practice advance, however, therapeutic standards may change. For this reason and because human and mechanical errors sometimes occur, we recommend that readers follow the advice of a physician who is directly involved in their care or the care of a member of their family.

Manufactured in the United States of America on acid-free paper
95 94 93 4 3 2

American Psychiatric Press, Inc.
1400 K Street, N.W., Washington, DC 20005

Library of Congress Cataloging-in-Publication Data

Psychiatric case formulations / Len Sperry ... [et al.].
p. cm.
Includes bibliographical references and index.
ISBN 0-88048-367-9
1. Psychiatry—Case formulation. I. Sperry, Len.
[DNLM: 1. Mental Disorders—therapy. 2. Patient Care Planning.
WM 400 P973]
RC473.C37P78 1992
616.89—dc20
DNLM/DLC
for Library of Congress 91-21998
CIP

British Library Cataloguing in Publication Data

A CIP record is available from the British Library.

Contents

Preface

CASE FORMULATION has been a poorly defined core clinical skill in psychiatry and the mental health sciences. Yet this skill is required for passing oral examinations given by both American and British psychiatry boards. Furthermore, the ability to conceptualize and write succinct case formulations is considered basic to daily clinical practice. In fact, the shift to briefer, more cost-effective psychiatric treatments and managed care systems has positioned the written case formulation as central in the patient treatment and utilization review process.

In the past, the "art" of case formulation was part of the clinical lore "passed on" to trainees within one-to-one supervision and in case conferences in psychiatry residency programs. That there could be a "science" or rational basis for conceptualizing formulations was not imaginable until recently. Although adherents of the psychodynamic, behavioral, and biopsychosocial orientations continue to debate the proper form and content of a case formulation, these discussions have become more conciliatory in tone and convergent in focus.

In this book, we continue the discussion on case formulations by providing a forum for recognized specialists in four major psychiatric orientations to present a straightforward account of their perspective on conceptualizing and writing a case formulation. In addition, a written formulation and commentary on a common case, the case of Mr. A, is provided for each orientation. These formulations of a common case provide the reader a unique window into the heart of the formulation process and the similarities and points of convergence among the four different perspectives.

The four coauthors are practicing clinical and academic psychiatrists who are involved in psychiatry education at the undergraduate, graduate, and postgraduate levels. They have established themselves as researchers and writers in their respective specialties of psychoanalysis (J.E.G.), biological psychiatry (B.B.), cognitive-behavioral therapy (L.S.), and the biopsychosocial perspective (L.R.F.).

That four psychiatric clinicians and educators with widely differing theoretical orientations could get together and collaborate on a book of this nature is no small accomplishment. This collaboration in no way implies that our discussions and deliberations easily yielded to consensus. Actually, it took several months to arrive at an operational definition of case formulation that was acceptable to each of us. In many ways, our deliberations and discussions mirror the intellectual ferment that so typifies the search for convergence and integrative thinking in contemporary psychiatry. We do not have any illusions that our description and strategies for conceptualizing and writing case formulations represent the definitive word on the subject. Far from it. Much more needs to be done. But we all agree that the basic foundation has been laid.

The format of the book is quite straightforward. In an introductory chapter, we provide an overview of both theoretical and clinical practice issues concerning case formulations and present the case of Mr. A. Because of the clinical practice orientation of the book, theoretical discussion in Chapter 1 has been abbreviated. For readers who are interested in pursuing these theoretical issues in more detail, Appendix A, "Theoretical Issues and Psychiatric Formulations: For Those Who Are Curious or Who Need to Know," follows Chapter 1. In Chapters 2–5, we describe the basic assumptions and a method for conceptualizing and writing formulations for the psychodynamic, biological, behavioral, and biopsychosocial orientations, respectively. In each chapter, a concise written formulation for the case of Mr. A is provided, followed by a step-by-step commentary of the formulation. In Chapter 6, we highlight the similarities and points of convergence of the four orientations toward case formulation in terms of content, form, and structure. In Chapter 7, we provide two different practical, hands-on methods for conceptualizing and writing formulations, with step-by-step instructions and practice sheets. These approaches have been seminar tested on several groups of psychiatrists-in-training and at convention and grand rounds audiences of practicing clinicians. Finally, in Chapter 8, we provide a number of written case formulations for the most common case presentations in both inpatient and outpatient settings.

Above all, this book is intended to be a practical, hands-on manual. Because it explores an area of clinical psychiatry typically neglected by general psychiatry texts, this book should be of value to both the beginner and the advanced clinician. Psychiatry residents, medical students, psychiatric educators, and psychiatrists in managed care and other clinical settings can expect to increase both their understanding and skill in conceptualizing and writing effective case formulations. It will also be useful to psychology graduate students and interns, as well as to psychiatric nurses and other mental health professionals.

We wish especially to acknowledge the editorial support and encouragement of the American Psychiatric Press, particularly Timothy Clancy, former editorial director, Claire Reinburg, editorial director, and Carol Nadelson, M.D., editor-in-chief. A special thanks for the word-processing support of Dawn Stalbaum, Kim James-Jones, Marlene Bruegger, Nancy Pribanich, and Dianne Heitmanek.

CHAPTER 1

Psychiatric Case Formulations: An Overview

WHAT IS A PSYCHIATRIC FORMULATION? What is its value to practicing clinicians and clinicians-in-training? These are important questions that are being asked with increasing frequency.

A psychiatric formulation can be defined as a prescribed method for the orderly combinations or arrangement of data and treatment recommendations about a psychiatric patient according to some rational principles (Faulkner et al. 1985). In short, it is the clinician's compass, guiding treatment. As such, it should include a wealth of information about a patient yet be clear, concise, and usable in clinical practice. Traditionally, the development of formulation skills has been relegated to psychiatric education programs (Ross and Leichner 1986). Yet the performance of recent graduates on adequately and effectively formulating case material on their oral psychiatry board examinations suggests that formulation skills may be inadequately taught or learned. For example, a poll of examiners for the MRC Psychiatry Part II examination—the British equivalent of the American Board of Psychiatry and Neurology (ABPN)–Psychiatry oral examination—disclosed that 87% of examiners mentioned the candidate's inability to present a coherent formulation as their chief "reason for failure" (Reveley 1983).

Recently, it has become even more apparent that formulations are not valuable just for case conferences or training exercises. The shift to more brief, cost-effective psychiatric treatments and managed care systems is moving the written case formulation into a central role in the comprehensive patient treatment plan and utilization review process. There is ample indication that the ability to write succinct formulations is becoming a requirement for psychiatric evaluations, discharge summaries, and prior authorizations for treatment (Sharfstein and Beigel 1985).

In the past, the form and content of formulations were subjects of intense academic debate by adherents of different theoretical orientations

(Goldsmith and Mandell 1969; Helmchen 1983; Kline and Cameron 1978; Rusk 1969). Advocates of various orientations tended to focus on different aspects of case data and often drew different conclusions about etiologies and subsequent treatments. If more recent publications accurately reflect current clinical practice, however, this situation has changed (Faulkner et al. 1985; Lazare 1989b; Mackinnon and Yudofsky 1986; Napier 1988; Perry et al. 1987; Person 1989; Turkat and Wolpe 1988). Now these discussions are notable for their similarities and points of convergence, most likely reflecting the trend toward more integrative thinking in psychiatry (Abroms 1981; Beitman et al. 1989; Cameron 1953; Weiner 1975).

In this chapter, we introduce four major orientations pertaining to psychiatric formulations: biological, psychodynamic, behavioral, and biopsychosocial. We begin with an overview of different ways of conceptualizing formulations in terms of their components, theoretical assumptions and premises, and clinical hypotheses. We provide an overview of the four major orientations to psychiatric formulation. Finally, we conclude with the case of Mr. A, which will serve as a common case for discussion in Chapters 2–5.

Three Components of Effective Psychiatric Formulations

We believe there are three components of effective psychiatric formulations: descriptive, explanatory, and treatment-prognostic.

Descriptive Component

A descriptive component is a phenomenological statement about the nature, severity, and precipitant of an individual's psychiatric presentation. The descriptive component also aids the clinician in reaching three sets of diagnostic conclusions: whether the patient's presentation is primarily psychotic, characterological, or psychoneurotic; whether the patient's presentation is primarily organic or psychogenic in etiology; and whether the patient's presentation is so acute and severe that it requires immediate intervention (Weiner 1975). In short, the descriptive component is phenomenological and cross-sectional in nature. It answers the "What happened?" question. Although there are many different ways to conceptualize case data, for all practical purposes, the descriptive formulation lends itself to being specified with DSM-III-R (American Psychiatric Association 1987) diagnostic criteria and nosology.

Explanatory Component

The explanatory component attempts to offer a rationale for the development and maintenance of symptoms and dysfunctional life patterns. It is more etiologic and longitudinal than descriptive or cross-sectional in nature. The explanatory component answers the "Why did it happen?" question. Just as there are various theories of human behavior, there are various types of explanations (e.g., psychodynamic, cognitive, behavioral, biological, family systems, biopsychosocial) (Lazare 1989b). Clinical lore as well as research suggests that effective treatment is more a function of the clinician's understanding of etiology than of diagnostic nosology (Beutler and Crago 1987).

Treatment-Prognostic Component

The treatment-prognostic component follows from the descriptive and explanatory components and serves as an explicit blueprint governing treatment interventions and prognosis. Cameron (1953) called this an action formulation or working hypothesis. The treatment component addresses the "What can be done about it and how?" question; the prognostic component addresses the "How likely is it to happen?" question. As with the previous formulation components, there might be many ways to answer these questions.

You may say: "Well, I've seen and heard a lot of case formulations and many don't seem to have those three components." That has been our observation, too. Possibly the most common case formulations we have seen and heard involve only the first component. These descriptive or diagnostic formulation statements are usually framed in DSM-III-R terms. Dynamic and insight-oriented therapists are usually quite comfortable developing the second component and will frame their formulation statements in analytic, cognitive, or interpersonal terms to explain the dynamics of the case.

However well conceived such formulation statements are, we believe that they are necessarily incomplete and therefore are limited in their clinical utility.

Again, a complete and effective formulation will include all three components and can provide answers not only to "What happened?" and "Why did it happen?" but also to "What can be done about it?" and "How effective is it likely to be?"

For the past few years, we have been listening carefully to the verbally presented formulations of clinicians we consider mature and effective (i.e., their patients get better). We noted that almost universally, these clinicians include these three components in their formulations, irrespective of whether they consider themselves analysts, cognitive therapists, biological psychiatrists, or eclectics. Granted, the explanatory component would differ, but all three components would be present nevertheless. A careful perusal of written case formulations by recognized expert clinicians appearing in the professional literature in the past 5 years reveals this same phenomenon: all included these three components irrespective of their theoretical orientation (Mackinnon and Yudofsky 1986; Napier 1988; Perry et al. 1987; Person 1989; Turkat and Wolpe 1988). Thus we feel confident in making the statement that all three components—descriptive, explanatory, and treatment-prognostic—are necessary to specify an effective psychiatric case formulation.

Perspectives, Paradigms, and Psychiatric Formulations

How a clinician formulates a case depends largely on both the clinician's theoretical orientation and paradigm (e.g., psychodynamics, biological, behavioral, biopsychosocial) and on the clinician's perspective on knowing about problems in mental life (called epistemology).

McHugh and Slavney (1983) described two methods or perspectives for knowing about and approaching abnormalities in mental life. They are the disease perspective and the life-story perspective.

The disease perspective asks "what" types of questions and views the patient as the object of illness. Emphasized are symptoms, natural history of the illness, and the facts comprising a patient's suffering. This perspective discovers new truth by comparison and correlation and strives to develop a classificatory system of illness types. The legitimacy of this classification scheme is determined by the constructs of validity and reliability. This perspective emphasizes symptom description and classification, etiology, course of the illness, and prognosis. Not surprisingly, etiology is sought in biology: neurotransmitters, biochemical, structural, or other brain processes. In short, what is known is only what can be quantitatively measured. The emphasis is on form and objectivity. By implication, the clinician approaches the patient as an expert observer.

The life-story perspective focuses primarily on the mind rather than the brain. It asks the "why" questions about mental life. The goal of the life-story method is to construct a meaningful story about how certain symptoms emerge within a person's life experiences. This perspective seeks to understand the function that symptoms have in the psychological domain.

It deals with the patient as a subject and as a person with intentional behavior, affects, and thoughts. The story of a patient's illness appeals to the human passion for meaningful explanation and uniqueness. In short, this perspective emphasizes the uniqueness of the patient's construction of his or her mental life. By implication, the clinician approaches the patient more as a participant observer rather than as an expert observer.

Obviously, there are limits to both of these perspectives or epistemologies, and McHugh and Slavney (1983) suggested that these perspectives are complementary rather than mutually exclusive. These two perspectives relate, in part, to our earlier discussion of the descriptive and explanatory components of a formulation.

Both of these perspectives assume that the clinician's role is to formulate the case, and that the clinician's formulation is the goal of eliciting information from the patient and corroborating sources. But patients also have their own explanation or formulations for why they have the problems or concerns they experience. A series of studies on patient noncompliance with medical treatment has led researchers to conclude that treatment compliance can be enhanced by eliciting a patient's understanding of his or her problem—a patient's explanatory model—and his or her expectations of treatment and then negotiating a mutual treatment agreement (Blackwell 1976; DiMatteo and DiNicola 1982). A patient's explanatory model and treatment expectations have also been termed "the patient's perspective" (Meichenbaum and Turk 1983). It can also be designated as "the patient's formulation."

Lazare and Eisenthal (1975) and Meichenbaum and Turk (1983) pointed out a number of ways that eliciting and attending to a patient's formulation enhance psychiatric treatments. First, this communicates to the patient the collaborative nature of treatment. Second, this decreases the probability of resistance while increasing treatment adherence. Third, this can enhance the clinician's morale about the prospects for treatment. Whether a clinician believes that recognition of the patient's formulation is useful and a necessary part of treatment is in large part a function of some basic assumptions the clinician makes about the patient and the treatment process.

From perspective we now move to paradigms and their significance for psychiatric formulations. A paradigm is an explanatory representation of a theory that illustrates its functions and forms (McHugh and Slavney 1983). In psychiatry, paradigms represent the most comprehensive and current understanding of human behavior within each of the four major psychiatric orientations. Within the psychodynamic orientation, the dominant paradigm has become object relations theory (Perry et al. 1987). Within the biological orientation, the dominant paradigm is neuropsychiatry (Cummings 1990). Cognitive-behavioral therapy is recognized as the dominant paradigm in the behavior orientation (Fishman et al. 1988), as is the "split biopsychosocial" paradigm in the biopsychosocial orientation (Doherty 1989). Appendix A, "Theoretical Issues and Psychiatric Formulations: For Those Who Are Curious or Who Need to Know" gives a more in-depth presentation of these epistemological and paradigmatic issues.

Four Major Psychiatric Orientations

The purpose of this section is to introduce each of the four major psychiatric orientations to psychiatric formulation. We indicate their basic assumptions and premises about the nature of psychopathology and treatment and list four representative clinical hypotheses that characterize the orientation. The idea of specifying a limited number of clinical hypotheses that a clinician could utilize to review particular case material to develop a formulation was first proposed by Lazare (1973). The clinical hypotheses for the biological, psychodynamic, and behavioral orientations are modified from Lazare (1989a).

The Biological Orientation

The biological orientation represents the biomedical model in psychiatry. Biological psychiatry traces its roots back to Hippocrates, yet Kraepelin is primarily identified as its major proponent in modern times. The biological approach views psychiatric disorders as primarily organic diseases. Even in the absence of known etiology, the biological psychiatrist assumes that a syndrome with a predictable natural history identifies a disease entity (Rabkin and Klein 1982). The hope is that, in time, a specific biological etiology related to brain structure or function will be found for each psychiatric disorder (Cummings 1990).

In research settings, genetic causation, receptor functioning, and other biological markers are pursued. In clinical settings, psychiatrists utilizing the biological approach focus on etiology, pathogenesis, signs and symptoms, differential diagnoses, treatment, and prognoses. Symptoms are believed to be a manifestation of underlying dysfunction in structural, biomedical, or physiologic processes. Treatment is primarily somatic, when one is available. Medications, electroconvulsive therapy, diet modification, phototherapy, and even psychosurgery are such modalities. As does any other physician, the psychiatrist relates to the patient with respectful support but with appropriate distance to maintain objectivity.

Biological hypotheses include the following:

1. A patient's problems are understood, in part, as resulting from a known organic/medical disease.
2. A patient's problems are understood, in part, as being related to a concomitant physical condition.
3. A patient's problems are understood, in part, as a functional psychiatric disorder characterized by genetic transmission, biological markers, and/or responsiveness to somatic treatment.
4. A patient's condition is known to be treatable, in part, by psychopharmacologic agents or other biological treatment.

The Psychodynamic Orientation

Psychoanalysis has exerted considerable influence on American psychiatry. Beginning with Freud's original formulation, psychoanalysis has evolved to where there are currently three major paradigms: classical/ego psychology, object relations, and self psychology (Perry et al. 1987). Although there are differences among these three paradigms, there are a number of common themes. In the psychoanalytic approach, the etiology of neurosis and personality disorders is sought in developmental impasses, early deprivation, distorted relations, or intrapsychic conflicts. As a result of such psychological determinants, patients distort reality; experience anxiety, depression, or somatic symptoms; or act out (Mackinnon and Yudofsky 1986).

The goals of treatment involve resolving conflicts, developing healthier object relations and character change, and strengthening the ego. In therapy, the psychological meanings of affects, beliefs, and behaviors are translated into an adult perspective. Within the therapeutic alliance, the clinician is able to facilitate the patient's recall of painful traumas and memories that underlie the patient's dysfunctional ways of coping. In the process of working through, the patient gains insight and discovers more functional ways of relating.

The psychoanalytically oriented clinician may utilize psychotropic drugs as an adjunct to therapy. The clinician believes that even though symptoms may have been ameliorated, the patient will remain dysfunctional until character change occurs.

Psychodynamic hypotheses include the following:

1. The patient's problem can be understood, in part, as a result of central conflicts, distorted object representations, or narcissistic vulnerability.
2. The patient's problem can be understood, in part, through knowledge of the precipitating event or developmental crisis and its dynamic meaning.
3. The patient's problem can be understood, in part, by assessment of his or her character or personality structure.
4. The patient's condition is known to be treatable, in part, by psychodynamic approaches.

The Behavioral Orientation

With the exception of practitioners in psychiatry, behavior therapy commands considerable status among mental health professionals. Recently this has been changing, primarily because of developments in cognitive-behavioral therapy. Cognitive-behavioral therapy is a blending of traditional behavior modification or conditioning therapies and the cognitive therapy system of Aaron Beck, M.D., and his colleagues. Being a central treatment in the National Institute of Mental Health Treatment of Depression Collaborative Research Program (Elkins et al. 1989) suggests that behavior therapy has come of age in American psychiatry.

According to the conditioning paradigm, psychiatric disorders are classes of abnormal behaviors that have been learned as a result of aversive events and are perpetuated because they either lead to positive effects or because they avoid negative effects. Subsequently, therapy focuses on overt symptoms, since they are the problem rather than a manifestation of an underlying disease process or unconscious conflict. The cognitive-behavioral paradigm considerably expands this view of psychopathology (Dobson and Block 1988). The cognitive-behavioral therapies emphasize that cognitions affect behavior and that cognitions can be altered, resulting in changes in feelings, thoughts, and behavior (Lazare 1989a).

In the behavioral orientation, treatment includes a detailed behavioral analysis, a determination of the behaviors to be changed, a behavior contract, a selection of treatment methods, and a plan for evaluating specific outcome changes (Krasner 1983). Behavioral treatment techniques include desensitization, aversive conditioning, response prevention, anger management, assertiveness training, relapse prevention, and cognitive restructuring. Treatment strategies are individually tailored to different problems, expectations, and needs of patients. A collaborative relationship between patient and clinician is considered essential for effective treatment outcomes (Lazarus 1981).

Behavioral hypotheses include the following:

1. A patient's problems are understood, in part, as disordered thoughts, feelings, or behaviors that are casually related to antecedent events.
2. A patient's problems are understood, in part, as disordered thoughts, feelings, or behaviors resulting from reinforcing consequences of behavior.
3. A patient's problems are understood, in part, as a result of dysfunctional cognition or behavioral deficits.
4. A patient's condition is known to be treatable, in part, by specific cognitive or behavioral techniques.

The Biopsychosocial Orientation

The biopsychosocial orientation can be defined as a way of understanding disease and illness as a dynamic process involving the interaction of biological, psychological, and sociocultural factors. Molina (1983–84) suggested that there are four theoretical premises that further describe and differentiate the biopsychosocial model from other models.

The first premise is that illness is a dynamic process rather than a steady state. Just as living organisms are in a constant process of change and adaptation, the process of illness changes continuously as biological, psychological, and social factors interact. The second premise is that illness is not a single entity with a single etiology, but rather a process caused by the interaction of several factors. For example, depression is caused not only by object loss, neurotransmitter deficit, learned helplessness, or dysfunctional cognitions, but rather is the result of the interaction of several of these factors. The third premise is that a person is best understood in terms of indivisibility and wholeness rather than as separate entities of body and mind. General systems theory has been useful in articulating this and other aspects of the biopsychosocial paradigm (Molina 1983–84). From the perspective of systems theory, a person can be thought of as a unified living system composed of subsystems that exchange inputs and outputs of information among both the internal subsystems and other external systems. Examples of subsystems are biological, psychological, and social subsystems. The fourth premise involves the concept of vulnerability. Because of their interactions with each other, subsystems are vulnerable to be disrupted by the alteration of another system or subsystem. Such vulnerability or predisposition, whether it is related to genetics, familial factors, low frustration tolerance, limited social skills, or minority status, must be considered to understand the development of a disease process.

In the biopsychosocial paradigm, disease and psychopathology can be explained in terms of stressors and vulnerabilities of subsystems (Faulkner et al. 1985). For instance, changes in the biological or psychosocial environment can create stresses that interact with subsystem vulnerabilities to precipitate disruption in one or more subsystems. As the disruption spreads to other systems and subsystems, the stability of the person as a whole is disrupted. This generalized dysfunction is manifested by signs and symptoms.

In short, the biopsychosocial paradigm views disease and its treatment as a seamless web of biological, psychological, and social phenomena. Engel (1977) contrasted this paradigm with the biomedical model, which views disease and its treatment as reducible to biological factors, and with the psychosocial model, which ignores biological in favor of strictly psychosocial explanations. Although many generally endorse the biopsychosocial paradigm in theory, relatively few actually practice according to this paradigm. In actual practice, many clinicians adopt a "split" biopsychosocial perspective (Doherty 1989). Thus the more biologically oriented psychiatrist may accept psychosocial variables but emphasize the primacy of biological factors in real "disease." Similarly, the more psychologically oriented clinician may accept the need for the biological but actually practice from a psychosocial perspective. Perhaps this split biopsychosocial perspective is a necessary transition to the adoption of the systems view of the biopsychosocial paradigm envisioned by Engel (1980). As such, the split model is a convergence of the "radical" biological and the "radical" psychosocial perspectives.

Biopsychosocial hypotheses include the following:

1. A patient's problems are best understood in terms of multicausation involving biological, psychological, and sociocultural factors rather than a single etiology.
2. A patient's problems are best understood in terms of the patient's biological, psychological, and sociocultural "vulnerabilities."
3. A patient's problems are best understood as manifestations of the patient's attempt to cope with stressors given his or her vulnerabilities and resources.
4. A patient's condition is best treated with a multimodal approach that

is flexible and tailored to the patient's needs and expectations rather than with a single treatment modality.

We have now responded to the opening questions regarding the definition and clinical utility of psychiatric case formulations and provided an overview of the four major formulation orientations in contemporary psychiatry. In summary, Table 1–1 reflects the relationship between the three components of a case formulation and these four theoretical orientations. In Chapters 2–5, we describe these orientations in detail and articulate methods and formats for conceptualizing the psychiatric formulation.

The Process of Formulation: A Case Example

The case of Mr. A describes a relatively common psychiatric presentation. It will serve as the common case for Chapters 2–5 to illustrate the points of convergence and difference among four psychiatric formulations: the biological, psychodynamic, behavioral, and biopsychosocial.

The Case of Mr. A

Mr. A is a 42-year-old businessman who presents with complaints of loss of interest in his job, hobbies, and family over a period of 6 weeks. He acknowledges periods of profound sadness, reduced appetite with significant weight loss, insomnia, fatigue, and recurrent thoughts of death, but denies suicidal ideations. He denies any precipitants but does admit that his expected job promotion has not materialized.

Mr. A describes himself as unusually serious, conservative, and relatively unable to express affection. He also acknowledges trying to be perfect, needing to be in control of every social situation, and having an excessive commitment to work.

Mr. A indicates that his marriage has been worsening for several years and describes his wife as flighty, overemotional, and helpless under stress. For the past several years, she has been angry and distant and has declined to be involved sexually with him. Since the onset of his symptomatology, however, she has been solicitous and obviously concerned. Mr. and Mrs. A have two children (a 12-year-old girl and a 10-year-old boy) who appear to be doing well at school and at home.

Mr. A describes his family origin as troubling. His father deserted his mother when the patient was 12 years old, and, as the oldest child, he had to take considerable responsibility for younger siblings, as well as to work part-time while attending school. Mr. A's maternal grandfather committed suicide, and two maternal uncles were alcoholic. A paternal uncle died in prison after a long period of antisocial behavior.

Physical, laboratory, and neurological studies are negative. The DSM-III-R multiaxial diagnosis is as follows:

Axis I Major depression, single episode (296.22)
Axis II Obsessive-compulsive personality disorder (301.40)
Axis III No relevant current physical disorder
Axis IV Severity of Psychosocial Stressors: 3, with moderate stress due to marital discord
Axis V Current Global Assessment of Functioning (GAF) score: 52; highest GAF score past year: 67

Table 1–1. **Relationships between formulation components and theoretical orientation of psychiatric formulations**

Formulation components	**Theoretical orientations**			
	Biological	**Psychodynamic**	**Behavioral**	**Biopsychosocial**
Descriptive	Psychopathology is the product of psychobiological dysfunction.	Psychopathology results from intrapsychic conflicts, developmental impasses, or distorted object relations.	Psychopathology is learned as a result of aversive events and/or dysfunctional cognitions and is maintained by reinforcing events.	Psychopathology is a complex, integrative response to stressors as they impact the individual's biological, psychological, and social vulnerabilities and resources.
Explanatory	Symptoms are a manifestation of the underlying dysfunctional physiological process.	Symptoms are manifestations of unconscious processes and dysfunctional character structure.	Symptoms are manifestations of dysfunctional behavioral patterns and/or cognitions.	Symptoms are manifestations of the individual's attempt to cope with stressors given their vulnerabilities and resources.
Treatment—prognosis	The goal of somatic treatment is to normalize dysfunction or compensate for the effects of dysfunction in the most efficient, effective manner with the fewest side effects.	Therapy consists of resolving conflicts, strengthening the ego, and character change.	Treatment focuses on specific symptoms and maladaptive behaviors or cognitions based on a comprehensive assessment of their antecedents and consequences.	Treatment is directed to amelioration of symptoms and increasing level of functioning often through a multimodal approach that is tailored to the individual's needs and expectations.

Appendix A

Theoretical Issues and Psychiatric Formulations: For Those Who Are Curious or Who Need to Know

In psychiatry, the terms *paradigm, model,* and *theory* are often used interchangeably. Actually, the terms have different meanings. A *model* is defined as a pattern on which to base clinical practice. Although it is often used synonymously with the term *theory,* strictly speaking, a model is an explanatory representation of a theory (Walrond-Skinner 1986). A *paradigm* is a pattern or model that illustrates its function and form (Wolman 1973). Paradigm is a more inclusive and clinically useful term than either *theory* or *model.* Paradigm is also used in reference to the stages of paradigm changes or shifts. Kuhn (1970) described a four-stage cyclical theory of knowledge progression in a scientific field. In the first stage, called prenormal or pre-paradigmatic, individuals or small groups pursue investigations independent of one another. Because there is little or no cross-communication, each typically uses and develops idiosyncratic languages, methodology, and theories. In the second stage, called normal or paradigmatic science, rapprochement and cooperation occur, and the community of researchers and clinicians utilize a single framework or paradigm with a common language and methodology. This stage gives way to the third, the crisis stage, wherein new methods and designs yield results that are inconsistent with the common paradigm. This gives rise to a search for a new paradigm that can better encompass and account for clinical observations and data. As the crisis of the third stage is resolved by the adoption of a new paradigm, the fourth stage of resolution has begun. Throughout this book, we use the term *paradigm* with this connotation.

Among the many psychiatric theories and approaches in vogue today, we believe there are four dominant paradigms in psychiatry: object relations theory in psychoanalysis, cognitive-behavioral therapy in behaviorism, neuropsychiatry in biological psychiatry, and the split biopsychosocial paradigm of the biopsychosocial orientation. Erwin (1988) believes that the field is presently in the third of Kuhn's (1970) stages, with each of these paradigms competing for dominance. Since the adherents of each paradigm "function" in the second so-called normal science stage, however, cognitive dissonance is "tolerable," although there is a sense of uneasiness and a feeling that "change is in the wind."

There is considerable ferment today about the basic assumptions that underlie these dominant paradigms. Issues concerning basic assumptions about paradigms are the province of the philosophy of science. One of its branches, epistemology, is concerned with knowledge: that is, what is known, who knows it, and how it is known. There are different views of epistemology and each images the knower and the known and their relationship in different ways that greatly influence how a clinician thinks about and relates to patients.

There are three major epistemologies: objectivism, subjectivism, and constructivism (Rudner 1966). Objectivism makes a clear distinction between the knower and the objects to be known. Objects exist independent of the knower and can be known only by empirical observation and logical analysis. Procedural rules, such as the scientific method, "guarantee" that our knowledge conforms to the causes of reason and can be reproduced by other knowers utilizing the same rules. Theories of human behavior based on objectivism include the original formulations of behaviorism, psychoanalysis, and biological psychiatry. Objectivism is the predominant epistemology in psychiatry today.

Subjectivism assumes that truth and reality are reduced to what the knower sees, feels, and desires. Introspection is the primary procedure for generating knowledge, and procedural rules are not considered important. Not surprisingly, the science of psychiatry arose in reaction to this nonobservable, nonquantifiable, nonempirical, and nonreproducible epistemology.

Yet the objectivist position is not without its problems. Recent proponents of both the psychoanalytic and behavioral models have seriously questioned the value and legitimacy of the objectivist viewpoint. Kohut's (1977) self psychology is based a constructivist epistemology, and various behaviorists (Hampson 1988; Schwartz 1988; Woolfork 1988) have advocated for the adoption of a constructivist epistemology for behavior therapy. The self psychology approach of Kohut has the therapist assuming an insider's or participant observer's perspective rather than an outsider's perspective in the therapeutic relationship.

Constructivism espouses the belief that objective reality does not exist apart from the perceiver's construction of it. Constructivism holds that all human undertakings are value laden. The heart of this viewpoint is the recognition that one's hypotheses about the world cannot be directly proven. This does not mean that there is no place for science or a scientific basis for psychiatry. Rather, the constructivist holds that scientific hypotheses exist for two reasons: because they are useful in clinical work and because they have yet to be disproved or replaced by an alternative hypothesis. Scientific hypotheses are constructions that have utility in that they help us portray reality. More specifically, clinicians can never be objective observers, because they cannot be disentangled from the observations they make.

Constructivists place certain restrictions on how therapy is to be conceived. Issues of power and authority become obvious. The responsibilities of both patient and clinician must be considered and clarified, as well as the consequences of any actions involved in the therapy process. Thus therapy becomes essentially a collaborative enterprise.

A constructivist view of personality is that it is a product of the person's behavior and the manner in which that behavior is construed by others and by the self. In the constructivist view (Hampson 1988), personality is viewed as a combination of three equally important components: the known or the actor, the knower or the observer, and the self-observer. Traditional approaches to psychiatry have emphasized the study of what the actor displays to others. On the other hand, Kohut's (1977) self psychology has emphasized how the actor construes the self and how the actor is construed by others. Adler's (1956) individual psychology and Kelly's (1955) personal construct theory are constructivist orientations in that all three components are considered.

So what does this discussion of paradigm and epistemology mean for psychiatry in general and psychiatric formulations in particular? In the past decade, a number of mental health disciplines have reconsidered their paradigms and epistemologies. Major debates have occurred in family therapy (Coyne et al. 1982; Keeney and Sprenkle 1982) and in behavior therapy (Fishman et al. 1988). In psychiatry, McHugh and Slavney's (1983) *The Perspectives of Psychiatry* and Beahrs' (1986) *Limits of Scientific Psychiatry* have seriously questioned psychiatry's dominant paradigms and epistemology and have proposed alternatives. Furthermore, movement toward a more integrative paradigm in psychiatry will require a shift to a more constructivist epistemology.

References

Abroms GM: Psychiatric serialism. Compr Psychiatry 22:372–378, 1981

Adler A: The Individual Psychology of Alfred Adler. Edited by Ansbacher HL, Ansbacher RR. New York, Harper & Row, 1956

American Psychiatric Association: Diagnostic and Statistical Manual of Mental Disorders, 3rd Edition, Revised. Washington, DC, American Psychiatric Association, 1987

Beahrs JO: Limits of Scientific Psychiatry. New York, Brunner/Mazel, 1986

Beitman BD, Goldfried MR, Norcross JC: The movement toward integrating the psychotherapies: an overview. Am J Psychiatry 146:138–147, 1989

Beutler L, Crago M: Strategies and techniques of prescriptive psychotherapeutic intervention, in Psychiatry Update: American Psychiatric Association Annual Review, Vol 6. Edited by Hales RE, Frances AJ. Washington, DC, American Psychiatric Press, 1987, pp 378–397

Blackwell B: Treatment adherence. Br J Psychiatry 129:513–531, 1976

Cameron EA: A theory of diagnosis, in Current Problems in Psychiatric Diagnosis. Edited by Hoch H, Rubin J. New York, Grune & Stratton, 1953, pp 127–142

Coyne JC, Denner B, Ransom DC: Undressing the fashionable mind. Fam Process 21:391–396, 1982

Cummings JL: Neuropsychiatry: the paradigm shift. The Psychiatric Times 7:41, 1990

DiMatteo MR, DiNicola DD: Achieving Patient Compliance: The Psychology of the Medical Practitioner's Role. Elmsford, NY, Pergamon, 1982

Dobson KS, Block L: Historical and philosophical bases of cognitive-behavioral therapies, in Handbook of Cognitive-Behavioral Therapies. Edited by Dobson KS. New York, Guilford, 1988, pp 3–38

Doherty WJ: Challenges to integration: research and clinical issues, in Family Systems in Medicine. Edited by Ramsey LN. New York, Guilford, 1989, pp 571–582

Elkins I, Shea T, Watkins JT, et al: National Institute of Mental Health Treatment of Depression Collaborative Research Program. Arch Gen Psychiatry 46:971–982, 1989

Engel GL: The need for a new medical model: a challenge for biomedicine. Science 196:129–136, 1977

Engel GL: The clinical application of the biopsychosocial model. Am J Psychiatry 137:535–544, 1980

Erwin E: Cognitivist and behavioral paradigms in clinical psychology, in Paradigms in Behavior Therapy: Present and Promise. Edited by Fishman DB, Rotgers F, Franks CM. New York, Springer, 1988, pp 109–140

Faulkner LR, Kinzie JD, Angell R, et al: A comprehensive psychiatric formulation model. Journal of Psychiatric Education 9:189–203, 1985

Fishman DB, Rotgers F, Franks CM: Paradigmatic decision making in behavior therapy: a provisional roadmap, in Paradigms in Behavior Therapy: Present and Promise. Edited by Fishman DB, Rotgers F, Franks CM. New York, Springer, 1988, pp 323–362

Goldsmith SR, Mandell AJ: The dynamic formulation: a critique of a psychiatric ritual. Am J Psychiatry 125:1738–1743, 1969

Hampson SE: The Construction of Personality, 2nd Edition. London, Routledge & Kegan Paul, 1988

Helmchen H: Multiaxial classification in psychiatry. Compr Psychiatry 24:20–24, 1983

Kelly GA: The Psychology of Personal Constructs. New York, WW Norton, 1955

Keeney BP, Sprenkle DH: Ecosystemic epistemology: critical implications for the aesthetics and pragmatics of family therapy. Fam Process 21:391–396, 1982

Kline S, Cameron PM: I: Formulation. Canadian Psychiatric Association Journal 23:39–42, 1978

Kohut H: The Restoration of the Self. New York, International Universities Press, 1977

Krasner L: Paradigm lost: on a historical/sociological, economic perspective, in Pain and Behavioral Medicine: A Cognitive-Behavioral Approach. Edited by Fishman DB, Rotgers F, Franks CM. New York, Guilford, 1983, pp 23–44

Kuhn TS: The Structure of Scientific Revolutions, 2nd Edition. Chicago, IL, University of Chicago Press, 1970

Lazare A: Hidden conceptual models in clinical psychiatry. N Engl J Med 288:345–351, 1973

Lazare A: Clinical hypothesis testing, in Outpatient Psychiatry: Diagnosis and Treatment, 2nd Edition. Edited by Lazare A. Baltimore, MD, Williams & Wilkins, 1989a, pp 103–110

Lazare A: A multidimensional approach to psychopathology, in Outpatient Psychiatry: Diagnosis and Treatment, 2nd Edition. Edited by Lazare A. Baltimore, MD, Williams & Wilkins, 1989b, pp 7–16

Lazare A, Eisenthal S: A negotiated approach to the clinical encounter, I: attending to the patient's perspective, in Outpatient Psychiatry: Diagnosis and Treatment. Edited by Lazare A. Baltimore, MD, Williams & Wilkins, 1975, pp 141–156

Lazarus AA: The Practice of Multimodal Therapy. New York, McGraw-Hill, 1981

Mackinnon RA, Yudofsky SC: DSM-III diagnosis and the psychodynamic case formulation, in The Psychiatric Evaluation in Clinical Practice. Philadelphia, PA, JB Lippincott, 1986, pp 213–277

McHugh PR, Slavney PR: The Perspectives of Psychiatry. Baltimore, MD, Johns Hopkins University Press, 1983

Meichenbaum D, Turk D: Pain and Behavioral Medicine: A Cognitive-Behavioral Approach. New York, Guilford, 1983

Molina JA: Understanding the Biopsychosocial Model. Int J Psychiatry Med 13:29–35, 1983–84

Napier AY: The Fragile Bond. New York, Harper & Row, 1988

Perry S, Cooper AM, Michels R: The psychodynamic formulation: its purpose, structure and clinical application. Am J Psychiatry 144:543–550, 1987

Person JB: Cognitive Therapy in Practice: A Case Formulation Approach. New York, WW Norton, 1989

Rabkin J, Klein D: The biological therapies, in Treatment Planning in Psychiatry.

Edited by Lewis J, Usdin G. Washington, DC, American Psychiatric Press, 1982, pp 89–150
Reveley A: Why do candidates fail the MRC Psych Part II? Bull of Royal College of Psychiatrists 5:51, 1983
Ross CA, Leichner P: Canadian and British opinion on formulation. Ann R Coll Ply Surg Can 19:49–52, 1986
Rudner M: Philosophy of Social Science. Englewood Cliffs, NJ, Prentice-Hall, 1966
Rusk TN: Dynamic formulation. Am J Psychiatry 126:578–579, 1969
Schwartz GE: From behavior therapy to cognitive behavioral therapy to systems therapy: toward an integrative health science, in Paradigms in Behavior Therapy: Present and Promise. Edited by Fishman DB, Rotgers F, Franks CM. New York, Springer, 1988, pp 294–320
Sharfstein SS, Beigel A (eds): The New Economics and Psychiatric Care. Washington, DC, American Psychiatric Press, 1985
Turkat ID, Wolpe J: Behavioral formulation of clinical cases, in Behavioral Case Formulations. Edited by Turkat ID. New York, Harper & Row, 1988, pp 5–36
Walrond-Skinner S: Dictionary of Psychotherapy. London, Routledge & Kegan Paul, 1986
Weiner IB: Principles of Psychotherapy. New York, John Wiley, 1975
Wolman B: Dictionary of Behavioral Science. New York, Van Nostrand Reinhold, 1973
Woolfork RL: The self in cognitive behavior therapy, in Paradigms in Behavior Therapy: Present and Promise. Edited by Fishman DB, Rotgers F, Franks CM. New York, Springer, 1988, pp 168–184

CHAPTER 2

Psychodynamic Formulations

THE PROCESS OF CASE FORMULATION begins the moment the clinician hears from or learns about a patient. The initial contact, whether by telephone call from a prospective patient, referral from another professional, or a face-to-face meeting with the patient, family, or referral source, sets in motion the process of formulation. A clinician forms an immediate picture of the patient's appearance and of the patient's thinking, feelings, and behavior. The following illustrates this initial contact for both patient and therapist.

> Mr. B called on the telephone stating he had been referred for psychotherapy by a psychiatrist and was prepared to start. The psychiatrist suggested they meet to learn more about what the patient wanted for himself. At the first interview, the patient expressed disappointment that the therapist had not immediately accepted him for therapy. The patient's primary reason for seeking help was a significant work block that left him paralyzed to complete a major project. The patient began therapy.
>
> Early in the treatment, this patient deprecated the therapist, noting how he had not been definitive in the original telephone call regarding the patient's therapy. The therapist was accused of being vague and uncertain. According to the patient, the therapist probably did not know what he was doing. The patient portrayed his highly successful father as definitive, harsh, and physically strong. In the early material, he recalled his father calling him to the library to lecture. His father expounded on making a success through hard work, often being critical of the patient's attitude. The patient was competitive with his father, as he was with men in authority, but was frightened he would not measure up.

Early formulation, to be revised as work progressed, could be made in terms of this patient's perception of himself in relation to men of authority. The patient's dilemma seen in the very initial set of reactions to the tele-

---

In this chapter, the case vignette of Mr. A presented in Chapter 1 is used to illustrate how dynamic formulation works. If you have not read Chapter 1, you may wish to go back and read the vignette to be familiar with the baseline data for development of this dynamic formulation.

phone call was a wish for but fear of authority. One anticipated he would struggle with negative and positive reactions toward the therapist. Over time, in therapy, he would recognize that all men were not necessarily as dogmatic nor as impotent as he imagined. This, in turn, would lead him to explore more closely his self-image and self-esteem.

Case formulation is a summary of a series of clinical observations that serves as a preparation for therapeutic intervention. It is the process of linking a group of data and information to define a coherent pattern. It helps establish diagnosis, provides for explanation, prepares the clinician for therapeutic work, and provides for therapeutic prediction.

Psychodynamic formulation is derived from the clinical interview: a special two-party relationship in which the patient seeks help from the professional. The clinician is the therapeutic instrument, serving as a microscope to diagnose the problem. The conduct of the interview, the particular reactions of the clinician in this relationship, influence the conceptualization and outcome for the patient.

All psychiatrists, regardless of theoretical orientation, should be able to gather anamnestic, descriptive data about the patient's chief complaint; present illness; development; family, social, educational, and work history; medical status; and mental status. The psychiatrist must learn enough from the patient to make a phenomenological (psychopathologic) differential diagnosis—currently using DSM-III-R (American Psychiatric Association 1987)—formulate the case, and make treatment recommendations. It should be clear from the onset that it is not the intention to divide interviewing arbitrarily or artificially into biological, psychodynamic, behavioral (cognitive), and biopsychosocial components, because all must be considered. Rather, the goal is to show how a theoretical orientation—the psychodynamic one—determines how a patient is interviewed and how data are gathered, assembled, and then formulated. It is customary to prepare a psychodynamic formulation after the initial interview(s), which leads to a treatment formulation, plan, and prediction. Formulation, however, is a continuous process from beginning to termination.

Obtaining Data: The Dynamic Perspective

In this chapter, we begin with methods and then conceptualization, recognizing that there is a constant interdependence between how one obtains data and how one understands and conceptualizes the psychiatric interview. Dynamic formulation cannot exist without the data. (Suggested readings for case formulation and theory can be found at the end of this chapter.)

For the initial introduction of patient and therapist, it is useful for the clinician to adopt a standard greeting for the patient. It is best to use the surname (Dr. . . .) because this establishes the doctor-patient relationship. Exceptions to this rule can be made for children and adolescents, and sometimes in family therapy. To use first names implies a degree of intimacy and friendliness that is not appropriate. Shaking hands is part of the initial greeting, but for some this, too, implies intimacy. For clinicians who start with a handshake, it may well be the only time during therapy patient and clinician touch. Much will be learned from the response of the patient: the patient may be hesitant, shy, passive, or anxious with perspiring palms, or the patient may be assertive, aggressive, intrusive, and demanding.

The interview room is the environment for work. Each clinician determines the image to be projected. No matter how the room is arranged, it becomes a curiosity for the patient. How the clinician chooses to place chairs, the type of chairs, and the distance between them are significant. In general, it is helpful to be seated 8–10 feet apart, with chairs facing toward each other but at an angle so as to point out into the room. With this arrangement, patient and therapist can make eye contact yet retain the opportunity to look away. The therapist who sits upright behind the desk or is hovering above 5 feet away communicates a very different interview style, which, in turn, can lead to very different associations for the patient. The patient who is offered a substantially less comfortable chair or who is seated in a chair lower than the therapist often has a sense of inequality in the doctor-patient relationship. The manner of walk, talk, appearance, dress, and style are observed by the therapist.

Here is an example of the impact of physical intimacy by a trained therapist on a patient.

> For Mr. C, treatment began with serious concerns about the disintegration of his 4-year marriage. The patient's previous 8 years of psychotherapy with a female therapist in another city had been useful in helping establish relationships with women. At the conclusion of the first interview, the patient announced that he would hug the male therapist. The therapist, using his customary approach, stated it might be more helpful to talk about this. The patient clearly was pained, proceeding to announce his former therapist had given him an embrace at the conclusion of each session. He exclaimed it made him feel good and reaffirmed therapy was safe, no matter what he had said.
>
> A previously established pattern with the prior therapist offering the patient an embrace was extremely difficult for the current therapist to undo. He would complete his session, arise and embrace the clinician, regardless of the clinician's stated intention to talk. For the patient, hug-

ging provided a real "holding environment," which avoided working on his needs for intimacy. By acting out the wish with the therapist, the patient was able to avoid the meaning of the act.

Although speculation, it may be that unwittingly the prior therapist had used her position of authority, benevolence, and hope to help the patient vicariously. It may be that the prior therapist was unable to accept the responsibilities inherent in the job or else used the role of therapist in a simplified manner, failing to understand the responsibility. A psychodynamic perspective helps to avoid these mistakes.

The vignette shows the psychodynamic therapist helping a patient put into words his thoughts, feelings, and actions. In this situation, as long as the patient acted on the feelings, it would not be possible for patient and therapist to understand the meaning of the act and use it in a constructive manner. Thus the setting, conduct of the interview, and development of therapeutic interaction are essential ingredients for psychodynamic understanding.

For an initial interview, the clinician starts with the question, What brings you to seek help at this time? The clinician wants the patient to tell his or her own story. Some patients have difficulty articulating their complaint. The pain of sharing intimate experiences may be too great; for others strong defenses preclude discussion; and for others idealization or devaluation stands in the way. The clinician asks open-ended questions: When did it begin? Where were you when you first had that experience? What did it feel like? Who was with you at the time? Say more about those initial feelings. The clinician is requesting the patient to relive the details of the initial complaint and immediate history to make it come alive, "in vivo," in the office. The dynamic clinician is not interested in the recitation of the facts without feelings nor in the feelings without the facts. The therapist is interested in how the patient tells the story as much as what the story is.

A few leading questions to show interest and responsiveness may suffice. Here is an example of material with a substantially more troubled patient and the beginning of case formulation. Although not a typical patient for psychodynamic psychotherapy because of the severe psychosis, the patient's case is presented to illustrate that a dynamic perspective can be useful with very psychotic patients.

Mr. D starts his story stating he just admitted himself to the hospital today because he was hearing voices telling him to kill himself. Satan was telling him he should be punished because he had sinned against God. He wanted other people to know things like that really happened. After a brief period, the therapist inquired when the voices began. He described basic training in the Navy when he needed to get out because a security check would reveal his bad past. The therapist asked if he could talk about that past or whether it was too painful. The patient said it was too personal, but stated that he had sinned with younger boys.

As the interview progressed, the patient talked about being the youngest of seven children. His parents separated when he was 2 years of age. He lived with his mother and maternal grandmother until his mother died of blood clots to the heart, and he was placed in a home for disturbed adolescents. The interviewer inquired if he felt like hurting himself. The patient responded that Satan told him to punish himself. Then he commented rather blandly that 3 weeks prior he took a knife to his abdomen, stabbing himself repeatedly as he tried to go up to the heart. The patient wounded his spleen, liver, and diaphragm, requiring emergency surgery in a nearby hospital.

Here we have a seriously disturbed late-adolescent who decompensated during basic training in the Navy. From this vignette, the therapist knows that he has a seriously ill, acutely psychotic individual who may be experiencing a psychotic depression or schizophreniform psychosis. The therapist proceeds to obtain details to establish the diagnosis, including further identification of the symptom picture, details of mental status, and personal and family history.

The interview identifies directions; one can hypothesize that closeness with other men in the Navy stirred up feelings. Whether another man approached the patient or whether he had urges to approach other men is not clear. The work is to re-create the Navy barracks scene in excruciating detail, to reconstruct whatever occurred that was intolerable for this patient. But this must be done carefully so that the patient's sense of panic with men is not increased. We know that the patient felt overwhelming guilt because the situation re-created for him earlier events in which "they made me try something against a child." We do not know to whom the "they" refers. We can hypothesize that this patient's childhood, loss of father at age 2 and mother at age 10, left him with few good, stable figures for identification.

Initial formulation suggests an ego vulnerability, perhaps apparent from early adolescence and possibly biologically determined, which presents as a full-blown psychosis following the occurrence of a significant stress. The patient is incapable of acknowledging, bearing, or putting in perspective by either ordinary or neurotic mechanisms the affects associated with loneliness, sexual and dependency needs, and intense dissatisfaction. There is an external factor (fear of discovery at the time of the Navy security check), an internal impulse (a wish for strength from a man), and a need to be cared for. "Just as a deserted and abandoned child may come to refuse food, clothing, shelter and withdraw in protest and despair, so the patient avoids everyday relationships to protect himself against the unbearable pain associated with past disappointments in these areas" (Semrad 1969, p. 18). Psychosis is the pathologic extreme, revealing flaws in development that had previously remained silent. For this patient, the severity of the regression reveals he requires a sustaining relationship to survive. He evidences through his suicidal attempt that his trust in the world at the most basic level is absent.

This patient did not know what his body was feeling. Instead he tried to die, possibly to punish himself or to rejoin his mother who had died from pulmonary emboli. In the interview, we talk about the pain in his heart, translating actions into feelings that can be identified in his body.

The psychiatrist is physicianly in manner, but does not give advice, counsel, or lay on hands. If the interview encourages spontaneity, the patient will take the opportunity to gain a better perspective and orientation. The interview should elicit the patient's spontaneous statement of his problem, special external pressures coming to bear on the situation, the way the patient is responding to his illness, the impact of developmental factors on his current state, and his attitude toward the therapist (Whitehorn 1944).

Some Specific Psychodynamic Techniques

The psychodynamic approach to a patient described has both inductive and deductive components. Inductive approaches have as their basis particular observations and instances that are used to arrive at more general understanding and formulation. Relative neutrality and open-ended observation are consistent with an inductive approach. As can be seen from the preceding discussion, getting the facts from a patient depends on the therapist maximizing the patient's opportunity to tell it as it is. Deductive approaches arrive at hypotheses on the basis of previously accepted theories. Deductive reasoning tests a theory against the observations. Implicit in virtually all clinical interviews are certain hypotheses derived from a more general theory of behavior. It may be that theory was derived from data, but theory now shapes interview style and technique.

Although not always considered a part of the psychodynamic armamentarium, areas of particular interest to the clinician include knowing the last straw. Precipitants often involve loss or a sense of failure. These include real object loss, somatic distress, childbirth, job, menopause, retirement, failure to achieve, or perceived failures for loved ones. Many more subtle losses can occur, such as loss of money, power, prestige, material possessions, and self-esteem. The loss can leave a vulnerable person inundated with unbearable affect and the regression can be significant.

The ability of a patient to tolerate stress is manifest in the body. Semrad (1966; Rako and Mazer 1983) spoke and demonstrated the technique: a "tour of the body." The clinician asks the patient where the patient feels the pain. Does it hurt in the head, heart, chest, abdomen, legs, arms, or genitals? The affects of grief, loneliness, isolation, and depression are often accompanied by somatic distress. Bringing to consciousness the relation of the body to the mind is useful. Depression is a response to real or perceived loss, whereas anxiety is a response to anticipated loss. With anxiety, somatic symptoms are likely to include light-headedness, headaches, chest constriction or pain, palpitations, perspiration, abdominal distress, or restlessness.

Triangulation is a process that may have been described first by Whitehorn (1944), who noted that the clinician uses a process that is similar to a surveyor's triangulator. The therapist takes two statements of the patient and imaginatively constructs a third statement to which there could be logical replies. Then, if a series of these constructions seems to converge, the interviewer has a tentative idea about what it is all about. The therapist continually compares the subjective reporting of feeling with the event to achieve a more objective report. The goal is not to challenge the patient, but to help the patient understand. Another way to define triangulation is to imagine going to the corners of a room and looking at an object from each perspective, then asking questions or comments from each perspective.

In general, the therapist stays on the surface in the initial interview. It is all too easy for a patient to provide a formulation of the problem based on an intellectual explanation from the past. Although in fact there may be truth to the formulation, it is more likely than not that this will not help the problem. Often it is useful for the therapist to share stories to illustrate or confirm a patient's report. This is best done when the story parallels the patient's account.

Empathy is the ability to feel within oneself the way the other person does and to put oneself in the other person's position. To be empathic requires that a person have the ability to go from participation in the other person's life to observation. Psychodynamic formulation is dependent on the capacity of the therapist to be empathic, for it is a recording of much about another person's life as seen from the perspective of the patient. Unlike empathy, sympathy places a value judgment on the situation. To be sympathetic is to feel sorry for the person; we send sympathy cards, not empathy cards.

There are pitfalls to an overly empathic approach or overreliance on empathy. In some situations, what appears as empathy may have more to do with the observer than the participant. Identification with the aggressor, a process where one identifies with the aggressive components of another's life and takes on the aggression within oneself, can easily be mistaken for an empathic approach. Identification, whereby one internalizes parts of another, can also be confused with empathy. An empathic explanation can be used as rationalization for a course of therapeutic action. Premature empathic statements without details can be disastrous. Thus the therapist must use empathy but not confuse it with a series of closely related, but different, mental processes.

To assist in the process of formulation, the clinician watches for and observes transference reactions. If we define transference as the set of emotional responses and attitudes that a patient has to the therapist based on prior experiences with significant persons in the patient's life, then the attitudes and perceptions expressed and conveyed to and about the therapist say much about underlying issues. For this reason, the therapist does not want to gratify the patient too much, so that the patient can project thoughts and feelings onto the therapist. Countertransference is the emotional reaction of the therapist to the patient. McLaughlin (1981) described this as the therapist's transference to the patient. Self-observation (the ability of therapists to train the microscope lens on themselves) is an essential ingredient to formulation.

At the same time that the therapist watches for transference reactions, the therapist is building the working or therapeutic alliance (Greenson 1967; Zetzel 1970). The real relationship and the positive aspects of transference are seen as an important part of the initial interviews. As described by Zetzel, a split takes place, allowing the mature part of a patient's ego to join sides with the analyst. In addition, all those subtle components of the real relationship between patient and therapist—shared experiences, perceptions of the world, style, aesthetics, philosophy—bring patient and therapist a shared communication and responsiveness.

Useful techniques to gain detailed information for a formulation include, but are not limited to, detailed understanding of the last straw, touring the body to gain access to affects, triangulation, working on the surface, empathy, and transference reactions. The patient is the best teacher, and learning comes from paying attention to what the patient says.

Aspects of a Theoretical Basis for Psychodynamic Formulation

It is not possible in this chapter to do justice to psychodynamic theory, but it is useful to review certain aspects of theory because it provides the guide and superstructure for formulation. Readings on psychodynamic theory are suggested at the end of this chapter. The work of White (1948), Brenner (1974), and Meissner (1988) as well as review of the original sources have been used for this summary. Kluckholn and Murray (1955) wrote:

> Every man is in certain respects
> like all other men,
> like some other men,
> like no other man. (p. 53)

The subject of Freud's (1893–95) first case report, Anna O, was treated between the years 1880 and 1882 by his well-respected Viennese colleague Joseph Breuer. Anna O, a woman in her early 20s, suffered from a panoply of symptoms and signs. Her right upper arm and both legs were intermittently paralyzed and her muscles contracted; a persistent cough, convergent squint, and dreamlike states called "absences" were present. These symptoms and signs today would lend a DSM-III-R diagnosis of conversion and depersonalization disorder, just as in 1896 this presentation was called hysteria. As reported by Freud and Breuer, these symptoms and signs could be removed in hypnosis, not by suggestion but by getting the patient to recall experiences and painful affects that had immediately preceded the development of a particular symptom. For example, Anna O, under hypnosis, recalled her father was on his deathbed when she fell asleep with her right arm over a chair. She had a dream that a black snake was coming toward her father, but she tried to fend it off. She awoke terrified and freed her arm, which was over the chair and had fallen "asleep." Hastily she put her feelings behind least she fail her dying father.

Symptoms could be cleared by a "chimney sweeping" process, which traced the symptom's origin steadily backward and brought to awareness painful memories not previously available. At the termination of therapy, it was reported that Anna O was left with a strong sexual attraction for Breuer. This woman who was the epitome of modesty and kindness, who was unsuggestible and had no sexual life and had a monotonous family life allegedly fell in love with Breuer. According to some reports, Breuer found this situation highly unwelcome and rapidly left psychiatry to return to neurology, but Freud, instead, went on to modify this technique and explain why this love affair occurred.

Because not all patients were good subjects for hypnosis and not all patients progressed, Freud began asking patients to remember painful events, of which they were not immediately aware, while awake. This process of recalling events became the cornerstone of a new technique, psychoanalysis. Patients were instructed to report to him whatever thoughts and feelings came to mind no matter how trivial and inconsequential they seemed. The new method—free association—allowed patients to remember things that were not usually available. Later, Freud returned to the subject of Anna O's change in personality. He explained this in terms of transference that developed between Anna O and her therapist. The intensity of this imagined love affair would be called a transference neurosis because it had origins in earlier romantic attachments and transferred these latent desires to her therapist.

The topographic model (Brenner 1955, 1980; Rapaport and Gill 1959) was Freud's earliest approach to mental functioning. In this hypothetical structure, there are three forms of mental functioning: conscious processes; preconscious, where ideas are close to the surface but not available; and the unconscious. Repression is the primary mechanism for keeping unconscious thoughts and feelings from reaching awareness. Daily mental functioning is not always what it appears to be because unacceptable thoughts are repressed. Later, Freud would reformulate and reconceptualize the origin of neurotic symptoms, relying on an anxiety model, but at this time anxiety and neurotic symptoms emerged from the unconscious.

To explain forces driving the individual, Freud postulated a libido or life instinct. Toward the later part of his life and after World War I, Freud (1920) added a death instinct. The instinctual model of functioning states that instincts and their derivates, drives, are inborn. The human organism seeks to reduce drives, returning to a state of less excitation, homeostasis, and balance. Psychologists such as Harlow et al. (1971) and Olds (1956) questioned whether humans always seek drive reduction, and they demonstrated that curiosity and exploratory behavior are based on drive production and arousal.

From theories about unconscious process, Freud postulated a sequence known as the developmental or genetic model. During the first year and a half of life, the child's major interest is oral gratification. The child wishes to incorporate and retain food to reduce the hunger drive. Any number of problems occur in the mother-child relationship. It is postulated that disturbances in taking in, retaining, or expelling food can affect development. Fixations to modes of gratification or to objects occur at unconscious levels. Separation-individuation during the first 3 years of life involves the differentiation of the self from the love object (mother) and establishes a sense of reality and the course of ego development (Mahler et al. 1975). In adult life, a person experiencing stress can regress to an earlier period and point at which development was fixated; this regression can be associated with pathologic mechanisms, but it can also serve as a highly adaptive response.

The anal period, occurring from 1.5 to 3 years, is described as the stage in which pleasure and displeasure are associated with both retention and expulsion of feces. Toilet training becomes the battleground for expression of libidinal and aggressive instincts. Fixations in this period, as in all childhood stages, could be toward a particular object, toward a particular aim, or toward a particular mode of gratification.

The phallic phase and the oedipal phase or complex occur between the third and fifth years. Using the analogy to the Greek myth *Oedipus Rex,* Freud postulated that the little boy becomes attracted to mother and wishes father out of sight. But the boy suffers the fear of castration should he act on the impulse. Father may punish him, and mother will not gratify his desire. Resolution involves giving up these desires and forming an alliance or identifying with father. In contrast, for the little girl, castration ushered in the Electra complex, and she competes with mother for father's attention. For the girl, in classical analytic theory, she must initially give up mother to attach to father and then reidentify and cathect with mother. Oedipal and Electra complexes involve triadic relationships—mother-father-child—whereas earlier developmental periods involve dyadic relationships. Feelings involved in triangular affairs are seen as extremely intense. Love and hate are stirred up; rivalry, annihilation or death fantasies, and potentially pathologic fixations and perversions abound.

The "neo-Freudians" Horney (1937) and Fromm (1947) rejected the primacy of the libido and the libido attachment to the basic zones of the body. Emphasis was on the interaction of child with the significant people in the environment, especially the mother. The issues of parental interaction with the child—love, warmth, affection, and attention—were seen by these revisionists as important in development. The work of Erik Erikson (1950) placed the stages of development in a much broader context. With each stage of development, Erikson saw major tasks to be accomplished; he conceived of these as extending throughout life. While fixation and regression could occur, Erikson's focus was on the ability of the person to master tasks throughout life.

Psychoanalysts have questioned the developmental theory, especially with regard to the lack of data on early life experiences. The reconstruction of the past based on adult memories is colored by current realities and not just repression. Furthermore, adults simply cannot re-create the past with any certainty. In clinical work, Meyer and Black (1989) have reviewed how recovery of repressed events is hard to sustain "unless we understand the 'facts' to be what is currently operative and not what actually occurred."

Most psychodynamic clinicians do not subscribe to Freud's original idea that object relationships are determined solely by the instinctual unfolding of a predetermined development process. Object relationships involve the outside person as a valued entity and the interaction of the outside person with the subject. Mahler (1979), in discussions about the separation-individuation phase, noted the constant interchanges that take place between the person and the outside world, the introjected objects, and the unconscious.

The structural model is Freud's major construct of mental functioning. In this model, there is the id (representing the primary instincts or drives), the ego (representing the person's relationship with the outside world), and the superego (representing the shoulds and should nots of the world).

The id is the mental structure or hypothetical construct that represents the drives, primitive impulses, and the sexual and aggressive instincts. The ego establishes the relationship of the individual to the environment. The ego consists of such functions as perception, memory, adaptation, control, and intelligence. The ego deals with external reality, the ability for self-observation and analysis, concentration, initiative, and resolution of conflict. Freud described the development of the ego from a highly undifferentiated component of the id in which the ego initially used primitive methods of incorporation to take in objects from the outside world. The process of incorporation gave way to introjection and finally to more mature identification. The ego ideal represents that part of the ego that is concerned with gaining respect and acceptance and becoming what one wants to become.

The last apparatus, the superego, a part that is embodied with guilt, is formed out of the discipline or threat of discipline from the parents; it arises during the oedipal phase of development. Morals and ethics of society are transmitted by the parents and become part of the inner world of the child. Punishment or the threat of punishment socializes the child in his or her environment.

Psychoanalytic Hypotheses

The patient's problem can be understood, in part, as a result of central conflicts, distorted object representations, or narcissistic vulnerability. The dynamic operation of an individual is rooted in self-preservation or adaptation. In *Inhibitions, Symptoms and Anxiety,* Freud (1926) conceptualized anxiety as the real or imagined response to danger. There is traumatic anxiety, which is an automatic response to real danger, and there is signal anxiety, which is an ego function that alerts the ego to impending danger. Anxiety develops when there is conflict between the impulses of the id and the functioning of the ego or superego or conflict between these structures and the external world. Anxiety is an affective state characterized by a feeling of fright, a cognitive state that indicates one is in trouble, and a behavioral response characterized by fight or flight. As used by Freud, anxiety is a signal to warn the individual of impending danger or conflict.

Symptoms and signs of illness are a reflection of the anxiety reaction itself or a heightening of defensive processes or a breakdown of the usual modes of operation with symptom formation. The defense mechanisms developed by the ego are means by which it protects from anxiety. Defenses can be seen in hierarchical order. Primitive defenses of denial, distortion, projection, and avoidance often used in psychosis are means by which the ego preserves itself. Psychotic denial is the active process of refusing to acknowledge reality; in the extreme it can be manifest in catatonia. With distortion, the ego fools itself into believing self-flattering delusions to gratify unobtainable wishes. Distortion, such as neologisms and word salad, is used to keep people at a distance and is seen in hebephrenia. Projection, seen in the extreme in paranoid conditions, protects the patient's ego from self-criticism by placing responsibility elsewhere. Avoidance is the act of looking elsewhere and getting away from what hurts. All of these defenses can and are used by nonpsychotic patients, but in the extreme, when reality is no longer preserved, they are seen in psychotic states.

Neurotic defenses are attempts to gain support from other people. Anna Freud (1937) saw these "defense mechanisms" primarily as the ego's defense against the id in an operation to protect from the outside world. The obsessional defenses of reaction formation, doing-undoing, and isolation ward off impulses that hypothetically have to do with the anal period of development. The hysterical defenses of somatization and dissociation are seen as mechanisms to protect from genital impulses and desires. Repression remains the sine qua non for management of neurotic conflict.

The dynamic theory of neurosis postulates that the vulnerable person is overwhelmed by real or imagined anxiety, which previously had been controlled by usual defensive functions. A conflict within the individual is awakened by an external or internal stimulus. The neurosis, as expressed in symptoms and signs, serves to control, bind, and protect from unbearable anxiety. The neurotic conflict may be linked to unresolved childhood fixations and failures. Thus adult neurosis may be a repetition of unresolved issues of childhood.

The patient's problem can be understood, in part, through knowledge of the precipitating event or developmental crisis and its dynamic meaning. Although the nature of the stress seems trivial in some situations, the patient who has avoided reflecting on his or her own affective experience may suddenly be faced with enormous subjective pain. In more profound cases, the entire perceptual system is involved so that as the ego disintegrates the distinction of self from nonself—subject from object—is blurred and even lost. Current loss may re-create or represent to the individual earlier life losses and failures that were never adequately resolved. The reaction to loss or failure is well documented by Spitz (1965), Lindemann (1944), Bowlby (1969), and others. Denial, angry protest, despair, detachment, demoralization, and slow reattachment occur. For some, the natural process becomes delayed or turns to profound depression.

The patient's problem can be understood, in part, by assessment of his or her personality structure. Allport (1937) defined personality as "the dynamic organization within the individual of his psychophysical systems that determine his unique adjustments to his environment" (p. 48). Character can be seen as personality evaluated or judged. Habits, specific and general attitudes, sentiments, styles, and traits are all psychophysical systems. Freud pointed to the relationship of early childhood and adult personality traits. Reich (1949) introduced the term *character armor* to describe the relatively consistent personality traits that serve as protective mechanisms. According to Reich, these patterns are the subject of close scrutiny because they are resistances in the development of neurotic character formation. To make change and achieve understanding, it is necessary to examine these long-standing ways of interacting with the world, and this is accomplished primarily by analysis of resistance and transference.

Self Psychological Formulations

During the past 20 years, Heinz Kohut (1971) contributed a significant new emphasis with self psychology. Although rarely defined, the self is seen by Kohut as the center of initiative and identity. We cannot know the self per se: "only its introspectively and empathically perceived psychological manifestations are open to us" (Kohut 1977, p. 311). Kohut referred to the "I" and then said:

> We can describe the various cohesive forms in which self appears, can demonstrate the several constituents that make up the self—its two poles (ambitions and ideals) and the area of talents and skills that is interposed between the two poles. . . . and we can distinguish between various self types and can explain their distinguishing features on the basis of the predominance of one or the other of their constituents. (p. 311)

Kohut's (1977) central concept is the bipolar self. The child has the opportunity to develop a grandiose-exhibitionist self on the one hand and a cohesive idealizing parent image on the other. The grandiose self and the idealizing other are two poles of the self. For Kohut, structural defect in the self is attributed to genetic failures of mirroring and exhibitionism for the grandiose self and an idealized parent image for the idealizing other. Kohut's work shifts from drive and libidinal representations to object representations and their effect on maintaining a cohesive self. The healthy development of narcissism and object love versus its restriction and limitation determines pathology. For Kohut, narcissistic conflict occurs when stable self-representations are threatened. For the child, there must be the right amount of merging-mirroring and approving to establish the grandiose self and sufficient empathic response by a patient to produce the necessary idealizations. The person with a narcissistic personality disorder develops transferences of the mirroring or idealizing type (Morrison 1986).

Cooper (1986) stated that

> the psychopathology of narcissistic character disorder is, in Kohut's view, one of arrest of the development of adequate psychic structure—that is a deficiency disease. These failures in the development of self structure are prior to, and the source of, the apparent drive-related and conflictual materials that have been traditionally interpreted as the milieu of neurosis. (p. 135)

Psychodynamic Formulation: Mr. A

In Chapter 1, the case of Mr. A. was presented; the reader should have the patient in mind for this discussion.

Without more detailed history and data, it is difficult, if not impossible, for a psychodynamic clinician to develop a formulation specific to this patient. Formulation comes from the microscopic examination of the clinical interview and anamnestic data. The skeleton is present. Let us add some intestines, interstices, and flesh to go on the bones as we might have learned from the initial dynamic interview. We will give this patient a heart and head. We will assume more information is available than is presented in the initial vignette.

Case Summary Statement

Mr. A, a 42-year-old married businessman and father of two children, presents with complaints of loss of interest in his job, hobbies, and family over a 6-week period.

Eight weeks prior to seeking help, Mr. A was passed over for promotion at the Able Candy Corporation by the president, who promoted a woman from the marketing department to a merchandise position. Mr. A recalls little reaction on the day his boss informed him. With questioning, he remembers the following night awakening from a nightmare in which he had profound dread of being far away and lost. Shortly, he noted a lack of interest and many of the symptoms of depression. However, he sees no apparent reason for being upset, because he claims it did not mean anything to him to miss out on the promotion. He has a recurring thought to run away to an island in the Pacific.

Mr. A's work history is characterized by hard work, achievement, dedication to the company, and a self-righteousness and impatience with others. For example, he describes being critical of several workers who leave work early. He has recognized in himself occasional mild annoyance with supervisors and peers, but has never expressed this. At home with his wife, Mr. A maintains a distant, aloof, somewhat superior attitude. He shows little warmth, dependency, or affection. He is hypercritical of his children, fearing they will not perform. He seldom acknowledges self-limitations. Mr. A met his wife during his senior year of college. He was studying business, and she was in nursing school. This was his first girlfriend. His mother disapproved of his choice because his future wife appeared flighty, immature, and bossy. Secretly, they married 1 month after Mr. A graduated, but the marriage was not revealed until a year later, when his wife completed college. The early years of marriage were good.

Since he was 12 years of age, Mr. A has not seen his father, who left home precipitously, according to relatives, because of an extramarital affair. Mr. A remembers his father as somewhat tyrannical and critical of him and knows that his father was unsuccessful as a car salesman. From the day his father left, his mother has never uttered a word about him. There has been no contact with his father. His mother was overinvolved and intrusive, especially regarding his homework. She did not date or remarry, but held a steady job and maintained an active social life with female friends, despite the fact that she was mildly, chronically depressed.

Descriptive, Nondynamic Factors

From a descriptive perspective, Mr. A suffers a major depression. His loss of interest, profound sadness, reduced appetite, insomnia, fatigue, and recurrent thoughts of death meet criteria for a diagnosis of major depression. His family history is positive for chronic mild depression, but there is no clear evidence of alcohol dependency, suicide, or antisocial behavior. Further data are needed regarding the patient's medical history, alcohol and substance use, prior depressions, and any use of medications. This would be obtained as part of the clinician's initial interview. Careful assessment of suicide potential is required. The clinician will need to know whether the patient has had thoughts of suicide or any plans of suicide or has any lethal methods for suicide, such as guns or pills, readily available. Direct questioning about suicide is mandatory given the current situation. With his propensity for denial, it will require careful observation.

From a developmental perspective, Mr. A, at 42 years, is in the latter stage of adult "settling down" or beginning of "mid-life." This brings with it a stage of hard work, job progression, and family life. The importance of enduring relationships and the establishment of characteristic modes of operation are expected during this period. Mid-life brings the perception that one has a limited future. The death of parents, relatives, and friends forces one to give up certain omnipotent fantasies and reassess reality and one's capabilities.

Psychodynamic Formulation: Central Conflict and Core Issues

A classical formulation of the acute situation suggests that Mr. A had considerable ambivalence toward his boss. In the context of being passed over for promotion, Mr. A experienced anger, denied this, and turned his anger inward on himself, internalizing the ambivalently held object and experiencing this as a loss of self or self-esteem. He regressed to a more dependent position, seeking love from his wife, which reenacts an earlier oral-dependent or aggressive fixation. He suffers from an unresolved or delayed grief reaction.

A second formulation of the acute situation can be stated. Mr. A had a conflict between the need to be perfect and in control, and an underlying image of himself as weak, imperfect, and ineffectual. Depression is understood in terms of his profound disappointment in himself, inability to gain rewards from the boss, fear of exposure to his wife, and fear of failure in the eyes of his mother. He internalized his mother's expectations, but harbored substantial anger at her overintrusive demands. He pushed aside the issue of his father. Ambivalence and anger toward his father were well concealed. The focal conflict between a need to prove himself and fear of inadequacy, the ambivalence with which he holds objects, and his struggle to maintain independence are related to original conflicts with his parental figures.

In addition, predisposing personality characteristics contribute to Mr. A's situation. The patient frequently looked for support from male teachers, but seldom found a mentor. He experienced self-doubt, but hid this effectively at work. Falling in love and marriage were clearly positive experiences, although he often wanted to control the marriage. The ages of his children reinforce a fantasy that to leave is a solution, one that he experienced with his father. His recurring desire to be free and independent may represent an identification with his lost father and repetition compulsion.

With limited data, a definite personality diagnosis cannot be made, but there is evidence for obsessional trends. The style of operation involving hard work, self-criticism, distancing from people, competitive interactions, isolation of affect, and downplaying of emotional reactions through rationalization all point toward an obsessional personality. A degree of self-centeredness and narcissism should be kept in mind as well.

Thus this formulation based on the theoretical orientation and specific techniques of dynamic work takes into account the current situation; the meaning of that situation to the patient; and the patient's self-concept, style of operation, and history. It provides an explanation for the observations.

To apply concepts of self psychology to Mr. A, we might envision that if there is a strong narcissistic component to his problem, he will develop grandiose expectations and/or idealize the therapist. Both responses are seen as arising from empathic failures or deficits of childhood. One can conceptualize depression as a response to failed grandiosity. Mr. A's problem would involve his low self-esteem and continual need to please others. If he received inadequate mirroring, he would have suffered empathic deficits. Thus his current need for recognition may be an attempt to compensate for self-doubt and for ambitions that could not be realized (Perry et al. 1987).

Although there is a tendency for formulation to identify issues from a pathologic perspective, it is essential to keep in mind Mr. A's strengths. He is hard working and achievement oriented; he holds a steady job; he is a caring, concerned, and supportive husband; he assumes family responsibility; and he often showed affection in the past. He is interested in working out his problems.

Rationale for Formulation

In Freud's (1917) classic paper, *Mourning and Melancholia,* a distinction was made between the normal mourning process, where there was a real loss of an object or person, and melancholia, where there may or may not have been a real loss, but where there is a loss in self-esteem and worth. In mourning, there is the real object loss; in melancholia, it is an ego or narcissistic loss (Arieti and Bemporad 1978). For Mr. A, the failure to be promoted can be seen as a blow to his esteem, leading to a rather profound regression.

In melancholia, there is an ambivalently held object. The loss of object love is accompanied by anger. Rather than expressing this anger and turning it outward, the individual takes in and internalizes this loss, incorporating the lost object into the superego and then turning the anger on the ego or self. The libidinal object is experienced as a narcissistic injury to self-esteem. Abraham (1916), using a developmental model, saw pathologic depression as a fixation in the oral period of development and a repetition of early oral deprivation later in life, with regression to the oral-dependent or aggressive period. For Abraham there was a developmental predisposition for depression, so that conflict in later life initiated regression.

Bibring (1953) reconceptualized depression as a fundamental ego state:

> Depression can be defined as an emotional correlate of partial or complete collapse of self esteem of the ego, since it feels unable to live up to the aspirations (ego ideal, superego) while they are strongly maintained. . . . Depression represents a state of the ego. . . . an affective state, which indicates a state in terms of helplessness and inhibition of functions. (pp. 26–27)

The process used to formulate the case of Mr. A began with consideration of his acute situation. Careful analysis of the precipitant and his overall personality structure suggests that the core issue is his failure to live up to aspirations, which although originally related to his mother and lost father, were now heavily internalized. These aspirations for success met with real failure. The collapse of self-esteem was tentatively held together by defenses of denial, rationalization, and undoing. However, his obsessional personality structure was heavily burdened by the collapse of his ego. One would anticipate that without treatment, this man would experience significant inhibition in his work and home life. The feelings of helplessness, hopelessness, and worthlessness would prevail.

Formulation: Therapeutic Plan and Prediction

Intervention with an antidepressant medication, after appropriate medical evaluation, may be indicated. The drug of choice is usually a tricyclic, although some might recommend a new blocker, such as fluoxetine. A tricyclic (nortriptyline, desipramine) will be initiated at low dosage and titrated upward with awareness that therapeutic effect may not be achieved for approximately 2–3 weeks. At this time, hospitalization is not warranted, but it should be kept in mind. It is the author's opinion that regardless of the psychodynamic understanding of this illness, psychopharmacology should be considered.

A psychodynamic formulation helps to explain how Mr. A is likely to respond to prescription medication. Appreciation of this man's obsessional personality structure suggests he will experience difficulty with control, acceptance of his illness, and dependence on medication. He may be guarded, scrupulous, querulous, overconscientious, and obstinate. A therapeutic strategy based on this understanding will help to know how best to prescribe the medication, how to elicit the patient's cooperation, and how to obtain reports from the patient about his response. For example, the patient may become distrustful of the therapist and fear he is controlled. More than most, one would expect side effects to be troublesome for this man. The therapeutic stance, clarification, confrontation, and interpretation accompanying the prescription of medication, will be based on this understanding. In turn, Mr. A's characteristic response to these procedures will form a basis to confirm or deny dynamic hypotheses. Underlying conflicts and transference reactions will emerge as part of medication management.

Unlike cognitive, behavioral, or interpersonal therapy, psychodynamic treatment planning has not been standardized and is seldom codified into a specific set of instructions. Instead, the dynamic treatment principles based on an overall understanding of behavior have been applied. The first question to ask is, Does this man want help? It is useful to ask, What does he want for himself? Is he interested in understanding and potentially changing? Motivation for psychodynamic work depends on interest in talking about problems and willingness to expose oneself and take chances. Some patients expect clinicians to do things to or for them and do not wish active participation. It may be that Mr. A wants medications only. It is necessary to assess whether lack of apparent motivation is part of depression or is a resistance. If a product of depression, it may require that the clinician recognize that the patient will be an active participant in time; if it is a product of resistance, early confrontation and interpretation are indicated.

Initiation of treatment can be with a statement of the central focus. Some therapists suggest that this be made explicit to the patient (Malan 1976; Mann 1983; Sifneos 1972). For Mr. A, this might be stated in terms of his inability to deal with his desire to achieve and fear of failure. For example, the therapist might say, "I notice that repeatedly you indicate you work hard to make things good but feel you do not benefit and in essence are the loser." A more encompassing focus would connect these themes to the patient's lifelong need for approval and the unresolved loss of his father. One might say, "Your loss of worth is related to the rage you feel toward your boss and is also related to a long-standing feeling of loss (for your father)." Another statement of focus might be, "Your grief in the present situation is related to your struggle for independence and the anger you feel when you are not wanted." Whether or not the therapist makes explicit a central focus depends to some extent on whether the therapist believes such formulation will be useful to the patient at the onset of treatment.

An initial goal may be to help the patient acknowledge his ambivalence toward his boss and verbalize disappointment. Relief from depression is the target. Bibring (1954) suggested a number of techniques. Abreaction is a process of emotional reliving of the warded-off painful experiences. Manipulation in therapy is mobilization of the patient's resources in a constructive way. Bibring pointed out that much of the therapeutic experience in itself is manipulation. The therapist's friendly accepting neutrality represents a new experience in relation to parental or other images. Suggestion is used to overcome resistance, encourage new solutions, or go around conflict. Clarification and confrontation can be used to help the patient experience his dilemmas. These techniques recognize the importance of conscious thoughts and actions as well as the unconscious motivation.

Following what may be an initial period of symptomatic relief, subtle symptoms and signs and character patterns will emerge. The patient will begin work on the issues of ambivalence toward the current people in his life (boss, wife, children, woman who gained the job promotion). He begins to deal with the therapist in his more long-standing characteristic ways. He may be obsequious, praiseworthy, yet show up late for sessions, skip sessions, save important ideas to the last minute of therapy, or openly devalue the therapy. These reactions will represent life's ambivalently held objects.

Change is based on understanding that past unconscious conflicts are repeated in the present (Karasu 1989). Strachey (1944) stated that a mutative interpretation consisted of a patient becoming aware of an impulse toward the analyst and simultaneously the impulse being directed toward a primary archaic object. Today, few analysts or therapists ascribe to the perfect mutative interpretation and the need for a full regressive transference. Current interpersonal situations are compared with past experiences with primary figures using the techniques of confrontation, clarification, interpretation, and working through (Greenson 1967). For Mr. A, interpretations that focus on present conflicts as they relate to ambivalence toward parents, parental separation, and loss might be useful. For example, at an appropriate point, one might interpret that the patient has kept his wife at a distance lest he be engulfed by her, as he had been by his hypercritical mother. Interpretation of self-defeating behavior as it relates to his job, family, therapist, and past can be useful. As the patient's depression lifts, a decision can be made with Mr. A to explore longer-standing issues, relationships, and characteristic modes of interaction.

Holmes (1861, p. 7) wrote: "Medicine is as sensitive to economic, social and political influences as a barometer is to atmospheric density." This perception is as true today as it was 140 years ago.

The professional freedom to choose the length and depth of therapy may be restricted. In material presented thus far, neither the patient's ability to finance therapy nor the physician's participation in various heath care organizations has been considered. The patient most likely is enrolled in an insurance plan with limited visits or a managed health care plan or the treating psychiatrist in an industrial health care organization, which limits visits. Thus the therapist may conceptualize the patient's problems in terms of acute symptomatology and longer-term personality disorder, but practice will require short-term intervention. Many advantages to short-term work have been noted, including reduced financial burden, expediency of a direct focus, greater accountability, and potential measurement of outcome (Karasu 1990). Disadvantages include insufficient treatment, relapse of illness, and inadequate opportunity to work through the vagaries of a long-term relationship. The notion of repeated short-term therapy at crisis points can also be considered, hence a form of interrupted yet ongoing therapy.

Briefer Interventions

Mann (1973, 1983), Sifneos (1979), Malan (1976), and others have attempted to specify patients who could benefit from short-term work, but there is no standard method among these therapists. For Mann (1983), the central therapeutic issue is conceptualized as "the wish to merge with another, but the absolute necessity of learning to tolerate separation and loss without undue damage to one's feelings about self. . . . life consists of a never ending series of reunions, separations and losses" (p. 29). The therapist provides an empathic encounter, helping the patient tolerate and overcome separation anxiety from key figures. To accomplish this, Mann states the central issue early in treatment in such a manner that it conveys both the current situation and the chronic pain. For Mann, a time limit of 12 sessions is established and firmly held. He anticipates that the patient will experience in the therapy situation initial abreaction and relief and a positive transference period of reexperiencing of the ambivalently held objects, and then separation and termination. His method is empathic—clarifying and interpretive—but transference interpretations are confined to the termination phase of treatment. The therapist must show the patient how present anxiety about termination is a repetition of early life separations and must help the patient to a more positive internalization and resolution. Mann does not have specific selection criteria, but assumes that a patient will be motivated.

Sifneos (1972, 1979) identified two types of short-term work: anxiety-provoking short-term psychotherapy and anxiety-suppressive psychotherapy. Candidates for anxiety-provoking therapy must be of above average intelligence, have at least one meaningful relationship, be able to express emotion during the interview, identify a chief complaint, and be motivated for change. In the initial sessions, Sifneos aims at formulating the central dynamic in terms of a present unresolved oedipal conflict. Sifneos will state this central conflict explicitly to establish the working relationship. Burke et al. (1979) likened Sifneos's method to "a school teacher seeing through the excuses and alibis of his recalcitrant pupils" (p. 178). Oedipal problems are categorized by Sifneos as those who linger too long in attachment to the parent of the opposite sex, those who are encouraged by parents to remain attached, and those who experienced death or permanent separation.

Sifneos's goal is to help the patient work through this central conflict, and he relies on active early interpretations.

Malan (1976) and his British colleagues develop a central focus through extensive interviewing and psychological testing. Unlike Sifneos, there are relatively few selection criteria. Unlike Mann, a specific length of treatment or number of sessions is not firmly fixed. It varies from a few sessions to 50, but the number is established and stated to the patient at the onset. Malan does not inform the patient of the focus, but rather provides genetic interpretations early in treatment and establishes their validity by the patient's response. Malan focuses on interpretation that relates the patient's conflicts to the present, to the transference, and to the primary parental figures.

Alexander and French (1946) suggested the corrective emotional experience focused on the here-and-now situation for the patient. They recommended that the therapist act in a way that was significantly different from the manner in which parental figures had acted and were perceived by the patient. The therapist consciously acts in every way to oppose the patient's tendency to see the therapist as a parent from the past. This technique relied on role-playing suggestion, coaching, and manipulation of the transference. Criticism to this approach has been that it may increase idealization of the therapist and dependency on the therapist, fails to address underlying conflict, and provides only temporary relief.

In this chapter, psychodynamic formulation has been presented in terms of its theoretical orientation, methods, mechanisms for change, and treatment goals. The psychodynamic model has been applied to a specific case of major depression to illustrate its potential positive effects. For conceptual clarity, this has been presented from a traditional psychodynamic framework, with neo-Freudian, ego psychology, and self psychology providing more contemporary additions. The recent emphasis on short-term therapy has been reviewed and contrasted with longer-term therapy in the treatment formulation. Today clinicians rely on a number of conceptual models and treatment techniques. While eclectic approaches prevail, it remains useful to explicate basic principles. Therefore, aspects of dynamic formulation may be seen as parallel, convergent, or divergent from other formulations.

References

Abraham K: The first pregenital stage of libido (1916), in Selected Papers on Psycho-Analysis. London, Hogarth Press, 1927, pp 248–298

Alexander F, French T: Psychoanalytic Therapy: Principles and Applications. New York, Ronald Press, 1946
Allport G: Personality: A Psychological Interpretation. New York, Holt, 1937
American Psychiatric Association: Diagnostic and Statistical Manual of Mental Disorders, 3rd Edition, Revised. Washington, DC, American Psychiatric Association, 1987
Arieti S, Bemporad J: Severe and Mild Depression. New York, Basic Books, 1978
Bibring E: The mechanism of depression, in Affective Disorders. Edited by Greenacre P. New York, International Universities Press, 1953, pp 26–27
Bibring E: Psychoanalysis and the Dynamic Psychotherapist. J Am Psychoanal Assoc 2:745–770, 1954
Bowlby J: Attachment. New York, Basic Books, 1969
Brenner C: An Elementary Textbook of Psychoanalysis, Revised Edition. New York, International Universities Press, 1974
Brenner C: Metapsychology and Psychoanalytic Theory. Psychoanal Q 49:189–214, 1980
Burke JD, White HS, Havens LL: Which short term therapy? matching patient and method. Arch Gen Psychiatry 36:177–186, 1979
Cooper AM: Narcissism, in Essential Papers on Narcissism. Edited by Morrison A. New York, New York University Press, 1986, pp 112–143
Erikson EH: Childhood and Society. New York, WW Norton, 1950
Freud A: The Ego and Mechanisms of Defense. London, Hogarth Press, 1937
Freud S: Studies on hysteria (1893–95), in The Standard Edition of the Complete Psychological Works of Sigmund Freud, Vol 2. Translated and edited by Strachey J. London, Hogarth Press, 1955, pp 21–47
Freud S: Mourning and melancholia (1917), in The Standard Edition of the Complete Psychological Works of Sigmund Freud, Vol 14. Translated and edited by Strachey J. London, Hogarth Press, 1957, pp 243–258
Freud S: Beyond the pleasure principle (1920), in The Standard Edition of the Complete Psychological Works of Sigmund Freud, Vol 18. Translated and edited by Strachey J. London, Hogarth Press, 1955, pp 7–61
Freud S: Inhibitions, symptoms and anxiety (1926), in The Standard Edition of the Complete Psychological Works of Sigmund Freud, Vol 20. Translated and edited by Strachey J. London, Hogarth Press, 1959, pp 87–172
Fromm E: Man for Himself. New York, Rinehart, 1947
Greenson R: The Technique and Practice of Psychoanalysis, Vol 1. New York, International Universities Press, 1967
Harlow HV, Harlow MK, Suomi SK: From thought to therapy lessons from a private laboratory. American Scientist 59:538–549, 1971
Holmes OW: Current and Counter-Currents: Medical Science With Other Addresses and Essays. Boston, MA, Tichner & Fields, 1861
Horney K: The Neurotic Personality of Our Time. New York, WW Norton, 1937
Karasu B: New frontiers in psychotherapy. J Clin Psychiatry 50:46–52, 1989
Karasu B: Toward a clinical model of psychotherapy for depression, I: systematic comparison of three psychotherapies. Am J Psychiatry 147:133–146, 1990
Kluckholn C, Murray HA: The determinants of personality formation, in Personal-

ity in Nature Society and Culture. Edited by Kluckholn C, Murray HA. New York, Knopf, 1955, p 53–70
Kohut H: The Analysis of the Self: A Systematic Approach to the Psychoanalytic Treatment of Narcissism Personality Disorders. New York, International Universities Press, 1971
Kohut H: The Restoration of the Self. New York, International Universities Press, 1977
Lindemann E: Symptomatology and management of acute grief. Am J Psychiatry 101:141–148, 1944
Mahler M: The Selected Papers of Margaret S. Mahler, Vol 2: Separation-Individuation. Northvale, NJ, Jason Aronson, 1979
Malan D: The Frontier of Brief Psychotherapy. New York, Plenum, 1976
Mann J: Time-Limited Psychotherapy. Cambridge, MA, Harvard University Press, 1973
Mann J: Casebook of Time Limited Therapy. Cambridge, MA, Harvard University Press, 1983
McLaughlin JT: Transference, psychic reality and counter transference. Psychoanal Q 50:639–644, 1981
Meyer JK, Black DP: Ego psychology: some theoretical notes. Discussion group on ego psychology, New York, American Psychoanalytic Association, December 13, 1989
Morrison A: Essential Papers on Narcissism. New York, New York University Press, 1986
Olds J: Pleasure Centers of the Brain. Sci Am 195:105, 1956
Perry S, Cooper A, Michels R: The psychodynamic formulation: its purpose, structure and clinical application. Am J Psychiatry 5:543–550, 1987
Rapaport D, Gill M: The points of view and assumptions of meta psychology. Int J Psychoanal 15:153–161, 1959
Reich W: Character Analysis, 3rd Edition. Translated by Wolfe TP. New York, Orgone Institute Press, 1949
Semrad EV: Long-term therapy of schizophrenia, in Psychoneurosis and Schizophrenia. Edited by Usden GL. Philadelphia, PA, JB Lippincott, 1966, pp 155–173
Semrad E: Teaching Psychotherapy of Psychotic Patients. New York, Grune & Stratton, 1969
Rako S, Mazer H (eds): Semrad: The Heart of a Therapist. Northvale, NJ, Jason Aronson, 1983
Sifneos P: Short-Term Psychotherapy and Emotional Crisis. Cambridge, MA, Harvard University Press, 1972
Sifneos P: Short-Term Dynamic Psychotherapy. New York, Plenum, 1979
Spitz R: The First Year of Life. New York, International Universities Press, 1965
Strachey J: The nature of the therapeutic action of psychoanalysis. Int J Psychoanal 15:127–159, 1944
White RW: The Abnormal Personality: A Textbook. New York, Ronald Press, 1948
Whitehorn JC: Guide to interviewing and clinical personality study. Archives of Neurology and Psychiatry 52:197–216, 1944

Zetzel ER: Therapeutic alliance in the analysis of hysteria, in The Capacity for Emotional Growth. Edited by Zetzel ER. New York, International Universities Press, 1970, pp 182–196

Suggested Readings for Case Formulation and Theory

Psychodynamic Formulation

MacKinon RA, Michaels R: The Psychiatric Interview in Clinical Practice. Philadelphia, PA, WB Saunders, 1971

Meissner WW: Theories of personality, in the New Harvard Guide to Psychiatry. Edited by Nicholi AM. Cambridge, MA, Belknap Press, 1988

Nicholi AM: The therapist-patient relationship, in The New Harvard Guide to Psychiatry. Edited by Nicholi AM. Cambridge, MA, Belknap Press, 1988, pp 7–28

Roth S: Psychotherapy: The Art of Wooing Nature. Northvale, NJ, Jason Aronson, 1987

Sullivan HS: The Psychiatric Interview. New York, WW Norton, 1954

Tarachow S: An Introduction to Psychotherapy. New York, International Universities Press, 1963

Whitehorn JC: Guide to interviewing and clinical personality study. Archives of Neurology and Psychiatry 52:197–216, 1944

Psychodynamic Theory

Brenner C: An Elementary Textbook of Psychoanalysis, Revised Edition. New York, International Universities Press, 1974

Greenson R: The Technique and Practice of Psychoanalysis, Vol 1. New York, International Universities Press, 1967

Meissner WW: Theories of personality, in the New Harvard Guide to Psychiatry. Edited by Nicholi AM. Cambridge, MA, Belknap Press, 1988

White RW: The Abnormal Personality: A Textbook. New York, Ronald Press, 1948

Yankelovich D, Barrett W: Ego and Instinct: The Psychoanalytic View of Human Nature, Revised. New York, Random House, 1970

CHAPTER 3

Biological Formulations

FORMULATION IS A SUCCINCT STATEMENT that encapsulates the etiology, evolution, diagnosis, treatment options, and future prognosis for the patient's problem. It captures the essence of each person's predicament and offers an opportunity to transcend the descriptive parsimony of DSM-III-R (American Psychiatric Association 1987) by portraying a complete biopsychosocial perspective without adding axes to an overloaded schema.

Formulation may also be performed within the framework of a particular ideology or body of knowledge, be it biological, behavioral, or psychodynamic. This may seem antithetical to convergent biopsychosocial thinking but is a necessary task that illustrates a pedagogical paradox. Teaching is facilitated by considering the parts to a whole, even though such reductionism seems inconsistent with an integrated approach intended to stress systemic, nonlinear interactions.

Throughout the history of medicine, biological schemata have been part of almost every framework to understand and treat mental illness, although their significance has waxed and waned with philosophical and scientific change (Hunter and Macalpine 1964). The turn of this century marked a clear point of divergence between the proponents of descriptive and biological psychiatry and psychological theories of behavior. The former were epitomized by Thudichum, Kraepelin, and Greisinger, each of whom believed that psychiatric disorders were predominantly brain diseases. The psychological theories were represented by scientists of equal stature, including Freud, Adler, and Jung. Freud, however, also relied consistently on medical models and metaphors. His preference for psychological understanding was related as much to the limitations of contemporary technology as it was to ideological principles (Jones 1953, p. 395):

> We have no inclination at all to keep the domain of the psychological floating, as it were, in the air, without any organic foundation. But I have no knowledge, neither theoretically or therapeutically, beyond that conviction so I have to conduct myself as if I had only the psychological before me.

Interestingly enough, the biological-descriptive approach held sway in Europe, while the psychological-dynamic theories became increasingly influential in the United States. For a brief period, Adolf Meyer's psychobiological approach offered a tentative synthesis, reflected in the nomenclature of DSM-I (American Psychiatric Association 1952). By midcentury and DSM-II (American Psychiatric Association 1968), the pendulum had swung back in a more purely psychodynamic direction (Spitzer et al. 1980). Even while this was occurring, observations and discoveries were being made in neuropsychiatry that laid the groundwork for a paradigm shift in a more biological direction. These included the protean psychiatric manifestations of neurosyphilis, which were benefited first by fever therapy and finally by penicillin (Sirota et al. 1989). The psychiatric sequelae of viral encephalitis following the worldwide influenza pandemic also provided striking testimony for a brain-behavior link (Lishman 1978). Impairment of intellectual development and behavioral abnormalities in phenylketonuria demonstrated that such changes could be due to biochemical and not just structural lesions (Szymanski and Crocker 1989). These etiologic clues were coupled with therapeutic strategies, which, while poorly understood, produced benefits that could be explained predominantly in biological rather than psychological terms. Included were the effects of electroconvulsive therapy, insulin coma, lobotomy, the amphetamines, and the barbiturates (Kalinowsky 1984).

By midcentury, the basis for a more biological understanding certainly existed, but the dominant paradigm in the United States remained psychological. Biological etiology was still poorly understood, and the treatments were either drastic, selective, or relatively ineffective. As Thomas Kuhn (1970) pointed out, such an ideological plateau is customary when evidence is not yet conclusive enough to overwhelm resistance to a new paradigm, which comes from practitioners of the prevailing "normal science." In the last half of this century, four concurrent trends have pushed the pendulum strongly in a more biological direction. First came the serendipitous discovery of almost all the major categories of psychotropic drugs within a single decade (1950–1960) (Ayd and Blackwell 1984). Second, the shortcomings of American nosology revealed by the United States and United Kingdom cross-cultural diagnostic project provided an impetus toward the more rigorous descriptive and nonetiologic DSM-III (American Psychiatric Association 1980) method of classification (Cooper et al. 1972). Third, rapid technological advances in several areas facilitated brain-behavior understanding. These included recombinant DNA methods with gene mapping (Gershon et al. 1987), receptor assays producing more specific drugs (Snyder 1985), biological and endocrine markers leading toward improved diagnosis (Whalley et al. 1989), and scanning techniques that display both structural (magnetic resonance imaging [MRI]) and functional (positron-emission tomography) aspects of brain function (Andreasen 1989). Fourth, and most recently, has been the social and economic impetus for short-term, more definitive and cost-effective forms of treatment that has favored biological over psychodynamic interventions (Parker and Knoll 1990). Societal adaptation to these trends is epitomized by legislative mandates that certain psychiatric conditions (such as bipolar disorder) be considered medical diseases and afforded the same insurance benefits as other physical illnesses.

Whether or not the current state of knowledge amounts to a full paradigm shift remains debatable, at least in the United States. Contemporary texts devoted to neuroendocrinology (Donovan 1988) and psychopharmacology (Meltzer 1987) are certainly encyclopedic, but, as noted recently by a reviewer in the American Journal of Psychiatry (Waziri 1990), books with a descriptive or biological bent are still outnumbered by those with a psychodynamic or psychotherapeutic bias. Despite the increasing pace of biological discoveries, there remains vehement opposition and criticism of the "disease model" in psychiatric practice (Johnstone 1989).

Whatever the contemporary Zeitgeist and however dominant the biological paradigm may appear, the practical question is the degree to which a core of scientific knowledge is available and useful to psychiatrists in the everyday understanding and treatment of patients. Is there a body of biological information that illuminates formulation? As Lazare (1989) noted, a biological formulation can be made based on the extent to which the information gathered meets four underlying hypotheses or assumptions:

1. The patient's problem can be understood, in part, as resulting from a known organic/medical disease.
2. The patient's problem can be understood, in part, as being related to a concomitant physical condition.
3. The patient's problem can be understood, in part, as a functional psychiatric disorder characterized by genetic transmission or biological markers that may predict treatment response.
4. The patient's condition is known to be treatable, in part, by psychopharmacologic agents or other biological treatment.

It will be noted that three of these assumptions are basically explanatory, and two include treatment implications. Although the discussion that follows provides some evidence to support these hypotheses, it would be presumptive to claim proof. The brain is a sensitive and finely tuned but well-protected organ, and most of our etiologic theories remain just that. In the single diagnosis where DSM-III claims an organic etiology (primary degenerative dementia), our clinical criteria are still often inconclusive with regard to underlying pathology. In one study, a third of patients diagnosed with Alzheimer's disease failed to show the appropriate postmortem neuropathologic findings to support the diagnosis (Risse et al. 1990).

Efforts to demonstrate a structural or biochemical basis for the major psychiatric disorders have been arduous and exciting but remain frustratingly inconclusive (hypothesis 1). In schizophrenia, for example, recent attempts to demonstrate brain abnormalities have focused more on neuroanatomy and neurophysiology than on biochemistry (Mesulam 1990). Neuroimaging techniques have sometimes shown an increase in the size of the frontal and temporal horns of the cerebral ventricles and a decrease in the size of the hippocampus. The ingenious application of these strategies to study the brains of monozygotic twins discordant for schizophrenia has shown that some of these structural changes are probably acquired and not genetic (Suddath et al. 1990). In addition, the overlap between "normal" controls and schizophrenic patients is substantial, and the findings are not specific to schizophrenia but can also occur in Alzheimer's disease and manic-depressive disorder. Similar uncertainties exist in interpreting the findings based on regional metabolic brain activity. Studies have reported both hypometabolism of the frontal lobe and hypermetabolism of the left temporal lobe. The findings bear an exciting correlation to the clinical manifestations of schizophrenia, with the negative symptoms of the illness resembling the results of frontal lobe damage and the positive features likened to manifestations of temporal lobe epilepsy. Again, however, it is unclear whether such changes truly reflect the underlying etiology of the disorder or if they are secondary manifestations of ongoing behavior or treatment. A recent editorial on this topic (Mesulam 1990) drew the following conclusion:

> It is currently impossible to distinguish primary pathophysiologic processes from secondary epiphenomena or idiosyncratic observations from those that are universal. Chances are that schizophrenia is a disease of the brain, but it is unlikely that such a complex, multifaceted, and fluctuating condition could be caused by fixed damage to a single brain site or neurotransmitter pathway. (p. 843)

Despite this absence of conclusive evidence of a general nature, the author of the editorial makes a telling point with regard to the biological formulation of individual cases in our current state of knowledge and its relationship to the use of contemporary diagnostic schemata:

> The evidence strongly suggests that at least some patients with schizophrenia have detectable structural and physiological abnormalities of the brain. Item E of the criteria for schizophrenia listed in DSM-III-R, the inability to establish an organic factor, may need to be eliminated. Perhaps this will start a trend towards the total elimination of the term "organic" which is often a source of obfuscation and an obstacle to lucid differential diagnosis. (p. 844)

The relationship of psychiatric manifestations to concomitant physical conditions (hypothesis 2) is well accepted and has been repeatedly demonstrated. One review lists more than 50 physical disorders in different categories that may present with psychiatric symptoms (Kirch 1989). These include neurologic, endocrine, metabolic, toxic, nutritional, infectious, autoimmune, and neoplastic disorders. Almost half of our patients have undetected medical problems, and in about half of these there is a direct contributory link to the patient's psychiatric symptomatology or mental status (Hall 1980). The extensive literature on this topic is consistent and compelling enough to justify the conclusion reached by Jefferson and Marshall (1981) that

> there are few if any, psychiatric symptoms that cannot be caused or aggravated by physical illnesses. The nonspecificity of altered mood, behavior or perception requires a clinician to continually contend with the possibility that there may be an underlying nonpsychiatric disease process accounting entirely for or contributing to an apparent "functional" disorder. (p. 1)

In addition to direct biological evidence of causation, clinicians and researchers have been eager to discover diagnostic tests or markers of disease that would assist in classification or treatment choice (hypothesis 3). Such attempts have a long but frustrating history influenced as much by fashion and the theories of the time as by sound scientific evidence. Historical examples include mapping bumps on the head (phrenology), culturing the bacteria in patients' stools (intestinal autointoxication) and, more recently, measurement of urinary metabolites (the biochemical classification of depression) (Kirch 1989). Among the most consistent attempts to identify a biological basis for clinical conditions has been evidence of genetic transmission. Pedigree analysis and twin and adoption studies have provided sound evidence for the biological contribution to many psychiatric disorders. The application of this information to the formulation of an individual case, however, has relatively weak predictive power. The development of gene mapping technology (Gershon et al. 1987) may alter this by providing the means of identifying the individual's personal genotype, as is already the case for Down's syndrome. In Huntington's chorea, linkage analysis of the potential patient and of affected and unaffected relatives allows almost certain prediction of the likelihood for developing the condition (Brandt et al. 1989). Unfortunately, this is a disease with no treatment, and genetic screening is fraught with psychosocial problems. Findings in major psychiatric disorders have been tantalizing but remain inconclusive. Individual kindreds have shown linkage for chromosome 11 in bipolar disorder and chromosome 5 in schizophrenia, but others have not. The impediments to accurate conclusions from linkage studies are considerable, and real progress is unlikely until the genes themselves are isolated (Merikangas et al. 1989). Even then it is almost certain that in psychiatric disorders more than one gene will be implicated and more than one neurochemical or physiologic process is involved.

The list of putative biological markers and laboratory tests used in psychiatric practice is extensive and includes imaging, electrophysiology, endocrinology, biochemistry, toxicology, hematology, serology, and microbiology. Only a minority of those tests studied for research purposes have proven practical and useful in clinical practice, although others have certainly supported the significance of biological contributions to causation. Examples include polysomnograph studies of rapid eye movement sleep (Roffwarg and Erman 1985); the use of blood platelets to study drug binding and receptor sites (Kafka and Paul 1986); and the various endocrine techniques used to study the hypothalamic-pituitary axis, including dexamethasone suppression and the thyrotropin-releasing hormone test (Loosen and Prange 1982).

It is frustrating, however, to note the disappointing outcome of some earlier attempts at investigations intended to enhance biological formulation. For a brief while, there was excitement about the ability to categorize depression into biochemical subtypes that would influence choice of medication, but it is now clear that most patients respond equally well to drugs that alter norepinephrine or serotonin or that may share some as yet unknown common mechanism of action (Kirch 1989). Equally disappointing has been the failure of the dexamethasone suppression test to achieve widespread utility. Its sensitivity and predictive value fell to unacceptable levels when the test was used in less selected populations than those in which it was developed (Carroll 1985). It remains possible that such tests may be refined or may have a selected use in a particular context—the prediction of suicide risk is one such possibility. Another is the finding that a positive dexamethasone suppression test is correlated with a poor response to placebo, indicating the need for pharmacologic treatment. However, response is not coupled with benefit to any particular type of antidepressant (Peselow et al. 1989).

It is in the domain of treatment (hypothesis 4) that we have attained more conclusive data. The scientific rigor of the double-blind, controlled trial at least allows some certainty in statements about the specificity of treatment outcome compared with placebo response or spontaneous remission. For both methodological and ethical reasons, such control measures are seldom applicable to outcome studies of psychosocial interventions, and although alternative strategies exist, the results are often less conclusive or compelling (Strayhorn 1987).

What such studies have shown is that biological treatments make a consistent contribution to improved outcome in most of the major psychiatric disorders (Ayd 1984). The treatment of schizophrenia has been transformed by neuroleptics, contributing to widespread closure of psychiatric facilities. A majority of patients with bipolar disorder benefit significantly and for sustained periods with the use of electroconvulsive therapy, lithium, and a variety of antidepressants. New categories of compounds with more specific pharmacologic effects are beginning to appear. The anxiety disorders show more varied and less global benefits, although there is increasing evidence that patients with obsessive-compulsive disorder improve specifically with somatic therapy. In conditions with a clear-cut organic etiology, such as Alzheimer's disease or Huntington's chorea, patients presently remain unhelped, but our rapidly advancing knowledge of their pathophysiology will eventually yield specific biological remedies.

The quality of evidence garnered from clinical trials may be constrained by flaws or limitations in the methodology (Newcombe 1988), and however compelling the results, they sometimes fail to influence practice because of stigma and social prejudice. For example, although research evidence shows clearly that electroconvulsive therapy is effective, opposition to its use persists, perhaps contributed to because its mechanism remains unclear, although hypotheses abound (Fink 1990). A similar controversy surrounds the use of cingulotomy for refractory obsessive-compulsive disorder (Bouckoms 1990). In the field of antidepressant drug therapy, Paykel (1989) reviewed the relevance of the research literature to clinical practice and concluded that the former certainly illuminates the latter with regard to general effectiveness but only "to some extent" in relation to specific treatment choices for an individual patient.

As in the rest of medicine, knowledge about the patient is derived from two primary sources: the history and the examination or investigation of the patient. These provide us with the symptoms, signs, and markers of disease. These two sources of information will be examined to illustrate the part they play in revealing biological factors that influence each of the components of a formulation: explanation (or etiology), description (or diagnosis), and treatment choice and prognosis.

Explanation and Description

Information may come from both the patient and other informants, including relatives or care providers. The latter may be most valuable in patients whose memory, judgment, or insight is eroded by biological impairment of brain function. The topics of particular relevance to biological formulation are family history and the possible precipitants, natural history, and symptoms of the condition.

In obtaining a family history, much may be forgotten and repressed or its significance missed or denied. Elicitation of a family tree across at least three generations (grandparents to children), specific questions about particular conditions, and use of cultural metaphors (e.g., "nervous breakdown") may help (Baker et al. 1987). Comorbidity should be considered (e.g., alcoholism in affective disorder) and atypical features (which often breed true) noted. Polygenic inheritance, incomplete penetrance, and cultural plasticity ensure that family histories of mental illness are seldom clear-cut or dramatic except in special circumstances with rare dominant pedigrees, such as Huntington's chorea or sequestered subcultures like the Amish.

History taking may reveal a number of etiologic factors that indicate a biological component. Existing medical diseases and their treatments contain manifold causes for a change in mental status, especially in anxiety and affective disorders or delirium and more rarely in psychotic phenomena. Communication with the patient's primary care practitioner may prove invaluable. Cause and effect are often attenuated; a drug or disease may enhance the vulnerability to a psychiatric condition rather than being a single or simple cause for it. A 58-year-old, black, middle-aged bus driver whose hypertension had been controlled with reserpine for 10 years became severely depressed for the first time after his wife's death. His depression did not respond to grief therapy or antidepressants until after his antihypertensive medication was changed. Presumably reserpine, with its tendency to deplete catecholamines, had created a biochemical vulnerability. Until this was corrected, other usually effective treatments did not produce a response.

Information on use of street drugs or dietary substances (e.g., caffeine in coffee or cola drinks) that may mimic, provoke, or exacerbate a psychiatric condition, particularly an anxiety disorder, should be requested.

Multiple organic factors may contribute to a final psychiatric outcome. For example, an 82-year-old woman living alone developed an early dementia and as a result forgot to nourish herself properly, then became dehydrated, and finally developed pneumonia, followed by a delirium.

In relatively rare instances, an occult and previously undetected organic condition will manifest itself as a psychiatric disorder. Examples are legion and include thyroid disease, pancreatic carcinoma, and thiamine deficiency. At times the psychiatric presentation will be so textbook or classic that the underlying organic etiology is discovered only during routine physical examination. Sometimes, however, there is a telltale amplification of particular features. The patient with myxedema underlying a depression may have extreme slowing of cognition or lethargy. The man with depression and pancreatic carcinoma may have weight loss disproportionate to change in appetite; the palpitations of a woman with thyrotoxicosis may be unrelated to psychological triggers.

An often-neglected aspect to identification of biological features of a disorder is that illnesses with a significant biochemical component tend to follow a predictable course. They behave like other medical conditions with a more or less clear-cut onset and natural history. There is an obvious point at which the person's behavior differs from his or her customary self in ways that may at first be more noticeable to others. This distinction between what is new (Axis I) and what is enduring (Axis II) is important, but not always easy to make since personality features may also modify or amplify the manifestations of the primary disorder. A successful young attorney who had always been the soul of discretion began to make sexually provocative remarks at the office and spent his entire savings on a trip to Hawaii accompanied by his secretary. Knowledge that he had a sexually repressed childhood and an unsatisfactory marriage should not postpone treatment with lithium before he bankrupts himself, ruins his career, or further damages his marriage.

The fact that failure to distinguish between a new major disorder and its effects in amplifying preexistent personality traits can have a potentially disastrous impact is illustrated by the *Osheroff v. Chestnut Lodge* controversy (Klerman 1990). A physician was treated for 7 months as an inpatient with intensive individual psychotherapy. His condition deteriorated markedly but he recovered within a few weeks after transfer to another hospital and treatment with psychotropic medication. The expert testimony that followed during legal proceedings focused on the issue of whether or not certain behaviors reflected a narcissistic character disorder or were attributable to untreated major depression. There seems little doubt that medication was inappropriately withheld, and the case has been widely construed as illustrating a paradigm clash between psychodynamic and biological models. However, it can also be seen as an issue of opinion versus evidence, with a rigid adherence to only a single approach when both medication and psychotherapy would have been indicated either concurrently or sequentially (Stone 1990).

Symptoms play a vital role in indicating a biological etiology. Alterations in orientation and memory are the cardinal features of an organic condition affecting the brain. A 45-year-old woman was brought to the emergency room by her husband while on vacation with the history that she had been drinking excessively for several months. On the morning of admission, he had found her in the hotel room confused and complaining of a severe headache. The emergency room physician diagnosed alcohol withdrawal, but the psychiatrist determined that recent alcohol consumption had been modest, the onset of headache was sudden, and the confusion was disproportionate to other signs of alcohol withdrawal. A computed tomography (CT) scan revealed evidence of a recent intracranial bleed. In the absence of trauma, a diagnosis of cerebral aneurysm was made and confirmed at subsequent craniotomy.

Other Axis I conditions not categorized as organic disorders may also have core symptoms that are empirically associated with a response to drugs and linked to a hypothesized biochemical defect. In major depression, these are the features of a presumed hypothalamic-pituitary dysregulation manifested by "melancholic" symptoms, including anhedonia, sleep disturbance, loss of libido, anorexia, and weight loss. Among the anxiety disorders are the protean symptoms of autonomic arousal that have been treated for centuries as somatic in origin. In schizophrenia, the core feature is a breakdown of integration between thinking, feeling, and behavior ("intrapsychic ataxia"), which manifests itself in Schneider's first-rank symptoms that are frequently responsive to those drugs that block dopamine receptors.

Interpretation of somatic complaints is particularly vital to accurate biological formulation. Their presence may serve to obscure, amplify, or mimic a psychiatric disorder. In consultation to medically sick individuals, the complaints due to organic disease may be indistinguishable from the somatic manifestations of depression or anxiety. Only such cognitive features as negativistic ruminations, hopelessness, suicidal ideation, or unrealistic fears may indicate the accompanying psychiatric disorder. A previously independent, active 40-year-old business executive developed an unexplained cardiomyopathy that required intensive medical management. During a prolonged stay in intensive care, he experienced multiple complications, including deep vein thrombosis, pulmonary embolism, and renal insufficiency. Assessment of a possible depression was complicated by extreme daytime lassitude, nighttime insomnia due to pulmonary edema, and fears that there was no end in sight to his suffering. His cognitive state was judged appropriate to his predicament and improved dramatically when an individual team member was assigned to explain interventions, plan daily assignments, and plot a rehabilitative course to create "light at the end of the tunnel." This case also illustrates the difficulty of differentiating a major depression (obscured by symptoms of organic disease) from an adjustment disorder with depressed mood in a medical setting, where symptoms of demoralization may be secondary to a protracted stay and multiple surgical or medical interventions (Snyder et al. 1990).

The meaning of symptoms can be modified not only by the patient's bodily condition but also by the mind-set of the observer. We can all be blinded by our role as psychotherapists and by the seductive influence of psychodynamics. At times we need to be reminded that as psychiatrists we are first physicians and as physicians it is our duty "to physich." This imperative to seek out, identify, and treat the biological components of illness is part of our social mandate. Even those of us who believe firmly in this obligation may be reminded of it by our own oversights. A few years ago I was treating a young woman referred to me by an expert psychopharmacologist who had completed a thorough medical workup. Her atypical depression and somatic complaints yielded temporarily to medication, but since she also had severe developmental psychopathology that disrupted her work and marriage, we met weekly for psychotherapy. Engrossed in the dynamics, complacent with my colleague's workup, and seduced by the early response to medication, both I and my patient minimized and misinterpreted her deteriorating physical condition. When her symptoms worsened abruptly, she attended an emergency room and was referred to a neurologist, who called to tell me that my patient had multiple sclerosis. The patient was not angry at my oversight, and our psychotherapy continued, but its focus shifted from interpreting or ignoring symptoms to adapting and coping with them.

A difficult aspect of biological formulation is the accurate assessment of bodily symptoms in the somatoform disorders, particularly in patients with accompanying medical conditions. This may call for considerable clinical acumen since the fundamental task is to determine the degree to which disability is disproportionate to known organic disease (Blackwell and Gutmann 1987). Neurologists and internists make this diagnosis on the basis of discrepancies or inconsistencies between signs or symptoms and the known pathophysiology of the condition, but psychiatrists have the added responsibility of eliciting what primary or secondary gain exists to amplify suffering beyond what disease can account for. What irreconcilable conflicts or irresistible rewards have driven or seduced the patient into the sick role? A 52-year-old, devout, Catholic Puerto Rican mother of two teenagers developed a relatively rapid onset paraplegia for which the neurologists could find no organic cause. Careful history taking revealed the symptoms began 24 hours after her 15-year-old daughter announced she was pregnant and 1 week after her son was arrested for dealing drugs. Her husband, from whom she was separated, had returned home to help deal with the family crises and had assumed all household responsibilities as a result of her sickness. The presence of such dynamics, however, should not blind us to the fact that fully a quarter of patients diagnosed as conversion disorder subsequently develop a physical condition (Watson and Buranen 1979).

Whatever our hopes for the biological revolution in psychiatry, we remain far more heavily dependent than the rest of medicine on history taking. However, examination and investigation are becoming increasingly important and contributory to formulation.

Examination includes both the patient's physical condition and mental status. Psychiatry still suffers from the psychodynamic excesses of the 1940s and 1950s when our specialty abolished the internship and espoused a "hands off" approach to evaluation. As part of the tragic error of "demedicalization," as recently as 1975 only 7% of psychiatrists believed that a physical examination was indicated or useful (McIntyre and Romano

1975). However, of those who did their own physical examination, 94% found them useful in establishing the diagnosis. Even today the task of examining the patient physically on admission to the hospital is still too often delegated to unlicensed physicians or moonlighting medical students who may have little understanding of how occult physical illness can cause or aggravate the patient's mental condition. This absurd dualism will continue as long as our training programs perpetuate it. Recently I evaluated an elderly man about to be discharged to a nursing home with a treatment-refractory retarded depression. The internist who admitted him had missed the significance of his slow pulse, sluggish reflexes, and dry skin. The psychiatrist who treated him unsuccessfully with antidepressants had overlooked the abnormal thyroid function tests. After correction of his thyroid status and treatment with electroconvulsive therapy, the patient's condition improved significantly, and he was again able to care for himself.

Equally important are the nuances of the mental state that may indicate a biological component. These are mainly those impairments of cognitive function in orientation, memory, and judgment that can be elucidated by the Mini-Mental State Exam (Folstein et al. 1975). Because fluctuations in mental state are a cardinal feature of organic impairment, it is often useful to examine the patient more than once (especially in the evening, when "sun-downing" occurs) and to obtain information from the patient's relatives or care providers.

It is especially important for the psychiatrist to be aware of the cognitive and emotional changes that may be related to structural lesions in the brain (Solomon and Masdeu 1989). On occasion, particularly early in the disease process, these may provide important clues to localization or etiology. Lesions of the frontal lobe (Ron 1989) are especially prone to present in an insidious manner that may mimic psychiatric disorder, resulting in delayed surgical intervention, sometimes with tragic consequences.

In addition to history taking and examination, laboratory tests and investigations may also contribute to biological formulation in two ways. First, they help to reveal or exclude concurrent medical conditions that may be causing or contributing to changes in mental status. Second, they may provide diagnostic confirmation of the psychiatric diagnosis itself. Precisely what tests are ordered should certainly be influenced by such factors as the patient's age, symptomatology, medical history, and proximity of previous physician visits. It is customary to include urinalysis, a complete blood count (including folate and vitamin B_{12} levels), and tests of hepatic, renal, and thyroid function. Electrolytes, blood glucose, a toxic screen (for drugs or alcohol), and syphilis serology are also important. Coupled with a chest X ray and physical examination, such a panel is usually adequate to rule out the majority of potential underlying organic conditions or to reveal the more common toxic, metabolic, or nutritional causes for a delirium. An interesting challenge to indiscriminate broad-scale laboratory tests (White and Barraclough 1989) found that only thyroid function tests (in women), urinalysis (in women), white cell counts, and syphilis serology were justified by the frequency of abnormal results. Obviously the quality of primary medical care in the population screened is significant, and it would be unwise to extrapolate such results from one culture (in this case Britain) to all other cultures, particularly when medicolegal considerations may be operative (as is true in the United States). An electroencephalogram may also be helpful in the diagnosis of protracted delirium or in revealing epileptiform processes that sometimes contribute to psychoses. CT and MRI provide clinicians with increasing specificity in the diagnosis of dementia, and neuropsychological testing may be valuable in the localization of cortical lesions.

In today's cost-conscious climate, clinicians should be aware of the criteria for imaging techniques (Weinberger 1984). There is increasing evidence that MRI may reveal more detailed and specific pathology than CT in some conditions (Jordan and Zimmerman 1990). Of special interest to psychiatrists is the finding of subcortical white matter lesions in various forms of psychosis (Conlon et al. 1990; Miller et al. 1989). Recently my colleagues and I investigated three elderly patients with late-onset paranoid delusions who had relatively intact cognition. Each had an abnormal MRI that showed subcortical encephalopathy. Although this may be a chance finding between a common clinical symptom and a new sensitive test, it illustrates the exciting possibilities that new techniques may offer in understanding etiology and enhancing diagnosis.

More specific neuroendocrine tests such as dexamethasone suppression or thyrotropin-releasing hormone stimulation are probably best reserved for those treatment-refractory cases (Zohar and Belmaker 1987) where it may be helpful to establish an organic basis for the condition before initiating more aggressive treatment strategies, such as electroconvulsive therapy or combination chemotherapies.

Finally, it should be remembered that an increasing number of patients with AIDS may present initially with a psychiatric syndrome (King 1990). The central nervous system manifestations of this condition are as protean as those due to syphilis in an earlier era. Human immunodeficiency virus testing with appropriate confidentiality may therefore be indicated, particularly in individuals who are members of at-risk populations.

Treatment and Prognosis

Biological features may also influence choice of treatment and prognosis. Drugs are not equally effective across the spectrum of Axis I disorders; biological agents are most likely to exert benefit in those conditions with most evidence for a biochemical etiology (Blackwell 1975). Disorders that can be provoked by chemical means may benefit from them. Reserpine can cause depression, amphetamine can cause a reactive psychosis indistinguishable from schizophrenia, and lactate infusion will induce panic attacks. Benefit derived from drugs in these disorders is due to their *specific* biochemical action (as opposed to change because of placebo response or spontaneous remission). These two latter sources of improvement are ubiquitous but variable with regard to diagnosis. A finding from controlled studies is that patients with obsessive-compulsive disorder show virtually no placebo response, so that although benefit from the active agent is seldom dramatic and often incomplete, it is always specific (Thoren et al. 1980). The elderly, on the other hand, who may be isolated and lonely, often display a large nonspecific response to low dosages of safe drugs that are little more than rational placebos. Patients with medical conditions tend to respond poorly to antidepressants, are often sensitive to side effects, and show little specific or nonspecific improvement. The use and outcome of medications in personality disorders are colored by the condition. Dependent patients may be difficult to wean; aggressive people may become disinhibited; and borderline patients will react to drugs as they do to people, with alternating idealization (a wonder drug) or disparagement (terrible side effects).

Beyond these broad generalizations, psychiatry finds itself at a disadvantage relative to the rest of medicine. There is no solid evidence for treatment specificity when selecting among drugs in a particular category to treat a defined Axis I disorder (Paykel 1989). For example, all antidepressants irrespective of their mechanism of action are equally effective and attain a comparable 70%–80% good outcome when given to a large, heterogeneous group of depressed individuals. The search for a specific responder to monoamine oxidase inhibitors has lasted for 30 years with results similar to the search for the Loch Ness monster—reliable observers report infrequent sightings but each describes something different (Blackwell 1986). More confusing still is the fact that drugs called antidepressants can benefit diverse conditions, such as chronic pain, enuresis, and panic disorder, often independent of a consistent improvement in affect (Blackwell 1987).

Faced with this lack of treatment specificity relative to the clinical syndrome, the choice between drugs is often influenced by other features of a disorder. The most reliable is a history of response to a particular drug in a previous episode; not only may this predict the degree of response but also its rapidity and completeness. Less often available and supported by a slender research literature is the notion that the response of blood relatives may predict benefit in a proband. Recently I treated a young woman with an atypical bipolar disorder who responded well to lithium after 10 years of chaotic life on the streets. When her mother witnessed the improvement, she insisted that her husband, who had been treated for years with phenothiazines at another institution, also receive lithium. He too obtained considerable benefit, and both father and daughter, who share similar clinical conditions, are now well stabilized.

A second avenue of influence on choice between biological interventions is the need to match the side effect profile of the drug to the susceptibility of the patient. An elderly man with a large prostate may develop urinary retention on a sedative tricyclic compound; an older woman placed on phenothiazines may begin to display parkinsonism. The elderly in general are vulnerable because of their altered metabolism, concurrent medical conditions, and other medications with which psychotropic drugs may interact (Raskind and Eisdorfer 1978). At times, electroconvulsive therapy may be the safest option for such patients.

Choice among medications is also dictated by the experience of the practitioner and the logic that underlies sequential exposure to different drugs. "First-choice" medications have the seductive property of reinforcing the prescribing prejudice of the practitioner, since spontaneous remission and placebo response are added to the specific pharmacologic benefit (Blackwell and Taylor 1967). Subsequent exposure of treatment-refractory patients to second-choice agents or augmentation protocols often follows a law of diminishing returns. An ideal "first-choice" drug is one that does not hamper subsequent treatment if it fails; fluoxetine (with its lengthy half-life) and monoamine oxidase inhibitors (with their prolonged enzyme inhibition) have obvious drawbacks. A major contribution of biological treatments to psychiatry has been the methodology of controlled trials, which can protect us from the referral biases and self-fulfilling prophesies of our own practice (Paykel 1989). Biological formulation is informed by the research literature as well as by individual experience.

Except on those occasions when they facilitate diagnosis, special investigations and laboratory tests provide little guidance for treatment choice in psychiatry. An exception is the use of plasma level monitoring for those drugs whose bioavailability and metabolism make such information useful in determining compliance, the adequacy of treatment, or its relationship to adverse effects (Kirch 1989). Lithium treatment and prophylaxis is undoubtedly the best example, but the use of blood levels may also be valuable in high-risk populations or treatment-refractory patients in whom the need to titrate medication carefully can dictate choice of a drug (such as nortriptyline) where there is a reasonably reliable relationship between plasma levels and outcome. Monitoring for blood dyscrasia is also routine in the use of carbamazepine and clozapine.

While prognosis is a part of formulation, it is a most uncertain art. In some of the brief reactive or schizophreniform psychoses, good outcome is linked to rapid onset, clear psychosocial precipitation, and affective features. In general, however, the heterogeneity of even our major classifications (Bleuler's "group of schizophrenias") and the multiplicity of biopsychosocial factors almost guarantee an unpredictable natural history in any individual, although it is true that controlled trials provide statistical blueprints within which to speculate about outcome. The likely length of any biological treatment is logically related to the natural history of the untreated and underlying biochemical condition (Blackwell 1975). But we have had biological treatments since the mid-1930s and effective drugs since the mid-1950s, so it is difficult to find untreated populations that would provide yardsticks. Age at onset, severity of symptoms, comorbidity, previous episodes, and psychosocial stressors may all enter the predictive equation, but often we have only a stereotype of good prognosis that applies to all interventions, biological or otherwise. Those likely to do well have a good premorbid personality; occupational, marital, and social stability; and a clear onset related to a defined precipitant. Nowadays one hardly needs to add that such individuals are also more likely to have good insurance. A counterpoint to the uncertain prognosis in psychiatric patients is that medical residents who rotate through our inpatient services express surprise at the good response of psychiatric patients to medications compared with the chronic treatment-refractory patients they commonly encounter on the medical floors.

The Case of Mr. A

The formulation of the case of Mr. A will be presented in two stages: first, a lengthy exposition that illustrates components with their underlying logic, and second, a pithy succinct synopsis that provides the essence of a model formulation.

Case Summary

Mr. A is a 42-year-old businessman who presents with complaints of loss of interest in his job, hobbies, and family over a period of 6 weeks. He acknowledges periods of profound sadness, reduced appetite with significant weight loss, insomnia, fatigue, and recurrent thoughts of death, but denies suicidal ideations. He denies any precipitants, but does admit that his expected job promotion has not materialized.

Mr. A describes himself as unusually serious, conservative, and relatively unable to express affection. He also acknowledges trying to be perfect, needing to be in control of every social situation, and having an excessive commitment to work.

Mr. A indicates that his marriage has been worsening for several years and describes his wife as flighty, overemotional, and helpless under stress. For the past several years, she has been angry and distant and has declined to be involved sexually with him. Since the onset of his symptomatology, however, she has been solicitous and obviously concerned. The A's have two children, a 12-year-old girl and a 10-year-old boy, who appear to be doing well at school and at home.

Mr. A describes his family origin as very poor. His father deserted his mother when the patient was 12 years old; as the oldest child, he had to take considerable responsibility for younger siblings, as well as to work part-time while attending school. Mr. A's maternal grandfather committed suicide, and two maternal uncles were alcoholic. A paternal uncle died in prison after a long period of antisocial behavior.

Physical, laboratory, and neurologic studies are negative. The DSM-III-R multiaxial diagnosis is as follows:

Axis I Major depression, single episode (296.22)
Axis II Obsessive-compulsive personality disorder (301.40)
Axis III No relevant current physical disorder
Axis IV Severity of Psychosocial Stressors: 3, with moderate stress due to marital discord

Axis V Current Global Assessment of Functioning (GAF) score: 52; highest GAF score past year: 67

Explanation

Mr. A's family history suggests a genetic predisposition to affective disorder, both directly on the maternal side with his grandfather's suicide and indirectly by comorbidity with alcoholism and sociopathy in uncles on both sides of the lineage. Other potential etiologic factors that need to be excluded by further history taking would include the absence of physical illness or the use of any medications and abuse of recreational drugs (particularly cocaine) or alcohol. In addition to facts obtained by history taking, these possibilities should be pursued with information from the patient's primary care practitioner and another family member who knows Mr. A's habits well. The negative results of the routine panel of laboratory tests (presumably including thyroid function) would also help to rule out any biological factors contributing to etiology.

Description

Two aspects of the illness itself support a biological formulation. The onset is relatively abrupt and marks a clear-cut change from a customary level of function. Second, there are features suggestive of melancholia that are often attributed to hypothalamic dysfunction. These include insomnia, weight and appetite loss, and anhedonia. Not mentioned but to be inquired about would be any changes in his sexual interest or activity (inside or outside the marriage).

Treatment and Prognosis

Outpatient treatment would be indicated by continued ability to work, absence of suicidal ideation, and support and involvement by his wife in medication management.

Since there are no previous episodes of illness, no family members treated for depression, and no concurrent physical illnesses or medications to influence treatment, the choice of an antidepressant would be dictated by need for some sedative properties to deal with Mr. A's insomnia. A tricyclic compound such as nortriptyline, imipramine, or amitriptyline would be selected, any of which could be subsequently monitored by plasma levels if response is problematic or if serious side effects occur. Before initiating treatment, discussion with Mr. A would determine his attitudes, beliefs, and concerns about the appropriateness of medication. Given his obsessional personality characteristics, some concern about the possibility of drug dependence might be anticipated. On the other hand, it is also likely that he would not be particularly psychologically minded and that an explanation based on a possible chemical imbalance would be appealing to him. Assuming Mr. A's concurrence with treatment, the benefits, side effects, and time course of response to medication would be explained. Immediate improvement in sleep would then be predicted, to be followed by a more insidious uplift in mood. A relatively low starting dosage would be given 2 hours before bedtime and titrated upward in small increments to obtain 6–8 hours of restful sleep with tolerable side effects. This dose would be maintained unless the predicted improvement in melancholic symptoms did not occur after 2–3 weeks, in which case the dose would be further escalated.

The prognosis given Mr. A would be good for this episode and somewhat more guarded for future affective illness. Of 10 individuals, 7 or 8 respond well to antidepressants, and Mr. A's history reveals several good prognostic features, including melancholia, a good premorbid personality, and a high level of social and occupational function. With affective illness, 50% manifests as a single lifetime episode, but future relapses would be more likely if etiologic factors remain unresolved. Both the duration of drug treatment and the likelihood of future relapses might therefore be related to the extent to which concurrent psychotherapy (psychodynamic or behavioral) and social change (e.g., divorce or job change) occur.

The average length of an untreated first episode of depression was about 6–8 months before there were effective treatments. Mr. A would be told that medication should be continued for at least this time period and that cessation of drug therapy would also depend on the extent to which life stress was reduced and his coping capacity had improved. When these criteria were attained, medication would be slowly weaned over 2–3 weeks to avoid withdrawal and treatment would be terminated after a further month or so of drug-free well-being.

The formulation of the case of Mr. A merits a final word of caution and comment that incorporates explanatory, descriptive, and treatment implications. Mr. A may invite the same kind of single-minded error illustrated in the *Osheroff* case (Klerman 1990; Stone 1990). Personality quirks are common, and nobody's life is free of blemish or painful incident. In this instance, the outstanding feature of the case is not the presence of such everyday occurrences, but the onset for the first time in mid-life of a new, severe, and incapacitating condition with no clear-cut cause. In the past, such illnesses were often considered "endogenous" and were typified by their rapid and complete resolution with biological treatment alone. It is distressingly simple to construct a web of psychodynamic speculation and, in doing so, to be seduced into withholding drugs while the patient is encouraged to "work through" his or her imagined predicament. Worse still, drugs may be pejoratively viewed as "trivializing the illness experience" or "stifling affect," with recovery dismissed as a "flight into health." Mr. A deserves better, and although he may benefit in the long term from psychological insights, he should never be denied psychotropic medication. The clinical criteria for different types of psychotherapy (cognitive, psychodynamic, or interpersonal) in depression have been well described (Karasu 1990), but it should be remembered that drugs alone would be the treatment choice in some cultures, that even if combined with psychotherapy they make the major contribution to variance in outcome for Mr. A's type of illness, and, finally, the rules of parsimony suggest that the simplest, most effective treatment be offered first.

The Biological Formulation

This 42-year-old, married, white father of two children has experienced a 6-week onset of his first episode of major depression characterized by melancholic features but without suicidal ideation. The family history is positive for affective disorder and comorbid conditions, but there are no other biological predisposing factors. Outpatient therapy with a tricyclic antidepressant is predicted to produce an excellent response based on good prognostic features, including premorbid personality and relative social stability. Prognosis for future episodes is more guarded and may be influenced by response to psychological interventions and social change.

Summary and Conclusion

In this chapter, we have considered biological formulation from several perspectives. First, we examined the degree to which technological advances as well as social and philosophical change have contributed toward a paradigm shift that attributes increasing significance to the biological understanding of psychiatric disorders. Next, we reviewed the extent to which existing knowledge supports the four basic hypotheses on which a biological contribution may be assumed. Finally, the way in which such knowledge is put to use in making a formulation has been discussed, both in general terms and then in specific relationship to the case of Mr. A.

References

American Psychiatric Association: Diagnostic and Statistical Manual: Mental Disorders. Washington, DC, American Psychiatric Association, 1952

American Psychiatric Association: Diagnostic and Statistical Manual of Mental Disorders, 2nd Edition. Washington, DC, American Psychiatric Association, 1968

American Psychiatric Association: Diagnostic and Statistical Manual of Mental Disorders, 3rd Edition. Washington, DC, American Psychiatric Association, 1980

American Psychiatric Association: Diagnostic and Statistical Manual of Mental Disorders, 3rd Edition, Revised. Washington, DC, American Psychiatric Association, 1987

Andreasen NA (ed): Brain Imaging: Applications in Psychiatry. Washington, DC, American Psychiatric Press, 1989

Ayd FJ: The impact of biological psychiatry, in Discoveries in Biological Psychiatry. Edited by Ayd FJ, Blackwell B. Baltimore, MD, Waverly Press, 1984, pp 230–243

Ayd F, Blackwell B (eds): Discoveries in Biological Psychiatry. Baltimore, MD, Waverly Press, 1984

Baker NJ, Berry SL, Adler LE: Family diagnoses missed on a clinical inpatient service. Am J Psychiatry 144:630-632, 1987

Blackwell B: Rational drug use in psychiatry, in Rational Psychopharmacotherapy and the Right to Treatment. Edited by Ayd FJ. Baltimore, MD, Ayd Medical Communications, 1975

Blackwell B: Antidepressant drugs, in Meyler's Side Effects of Drugs, Annual 10. Edited by Dukes MNG. Amsterdam, Elsevier Science Publishers BV, 1986

Blackwell B: Antidepressants as adjuncts in chronic idiopathic pain management. International Drug Therapy Newsletter 22:1–4, 1987

Blackwell B, Gutmann M: The management of chronic illness behavior, in Illness Behavior. Edited by McHugh S, Vallis M. New York, Plenum, 1987, pp 401–408

Blackwell B, Taylor DC: An operational evaluation of MAO inhibitors. Proceedings of the Royal Society of Medicine 60:830–833, 1967

Bouckoms A: Letter to the editor. Psychiatric Times, May 1990

Brandt J, Quaid KA, Folstein SE, et al: Presymptomatic diagnosis of delayed-onset disease with linked DNA markers: the experience in Huntington's disease. JAMA 261:3108–3114, 1989

Carroll BJ: Dexamethasone suppression test: a review of contemporary confusion. J Clin Psychiatry 46:13–18, 1985

Conlon P, Trimble MR, Rogers D: A study of epileptic psychosis using magnetic resonance imaging. Br J Psychiatry 156:231–235, 1990

Cooper JE, Kendell RE, Garland BJ, et al (eds): Psychiatric Diagnosis in New York and London. London, Oxford University Press, 1972

Donovan BT: Humors, Hormones and the Mind: An Approach to the Understanding of Behavior. New York, Stockton Press, 1988

Fink M: How does convulsive therapy work? Neuropsychopharmacology 3:73–82, 1990

Folstein MF, Folstein S, McHugh PR: Mini-Mental State: a practical guide for grading the cognitive state of patients for the clinician. J Psychiatr Res 12:189–194, 1975

Gershon ES, Merrill CR, Goldin LR, et al: The role of molecular genetics in psychiatry. Biol Psychiatry 22:1388–1405, 1987

Hall RCW (ed): Psychiatric Presentations of Medical Illness. New York, Spectrum Publications, 1980

Hunter R, Macalpine I (eds): Three Hundred Years of Psychiatry. London, Oxford University Press, 1964

Jefferson JW, Marshall R: Neuropsychiatric Features of Medical Disorders. New York, Plenum, 1981

Johnstone L: Users and Abusers of Psychiatry: A Critical Look at Traditional Psychiatric Practice. London, Routledge, 1989

Jones E: The Life and World of Sigmund Freud, Vol 1. New York, Basic Books, 1953

Jordan BD, Zimmerman RD: Computed tomography and magnetic resonance imaging in boxers. JAMA 263:1670–1674, 1990

Kafka MS, Paul SM: Platelet α_2 adrenergic receptors in depression. Arch Gen Psychiatry 43:91–95, 1986

Kuhn T: The Structure of Scientific Revolution. Chicago, IL, University of Chicago Press, 1970

Kalinowsky LB: Biological psychiatric treatments preceding pharmacotherapy, in Discoveries in Biological Psychiatry. Edited by Ayd F, Blackwell B. Baltimore, MD, Waverly Press, 1984, pp 59–67

Karasu TB: Toward a clinical model of psychotherapy for depression, II: an integrative and selective treatment approach. Am J Psychiatry 147:269–278, 1990

King MB: Psychological aspects of HIV infection and AIDS. Br J Psychiatry 156:151–156, 1990

Kirch DC: Medical assessment and laboratory testing in psychiatry, in Comprehensive Textbook of Psychiatry. Edited by Kaplan HI, Sadock BJ. Baltimore, MD, Williams & Wilkins, 1989, pp 525–533

Klerman GL: The psychiatric patient's right to effective treatment: implications of Osheroff v. Chestnut Lodge. Am J Psychiatry 147:409–418, 1990

Lazare A: A multidimensional approach to psychopathology, in Outpatient Psychiatry Diagnosis and Treatment, 2nd Edition. Edited by Lazare A. Baltimore, MD, Williams & Wilkins, 1989, pp 7–16

Lishman WA: Organic Psychiatry. London, Blackwell Scientific Publications, 1978

Loosen PT, Prange AJ: Serum thyrotropin response to thyrotropin releasing hormone in psychiatric patients: a review. Am J Psychiatry 139:405–412, 1982

McIntyre S, Romano J: Is there a stethoscope in the house (and is it used)? Arch Gen Psychiatry 34:1147–1151, 1975

Meltzer HY: Psychopharmacology: The Third Generation of Progress. New York, Raven, 1987

Merikangas KR, Spence MA, Kupfer DJ: Linkage studies of bipolar disorder: methodologic and analytic issues: report of MacArthur Foundation Workshop on Linkage and Clinical Features in Affective Disorders. Arch Gen Psychiatry 46:1137–1141, 1989

Mesulam MM: Schizophrenia and the brain. N Engl J Med 322:842–844, 1990

Miller BL, Lesser IM, Boone K, et al: Brain white matter lesions and psychoses. Br J Psychiatry 155:73–78, 1989

Newcombe RG: Evaluation of treatment effectiveness in psychiatric research. Br J Psychiatry 152:696–697, 1988

Parker SP, Knoll JL: Partial hospitalization: an update. Am J Psychiatry 147:156–160, 1990

Paykel ES: Treatment of depression: the relevance of research for clinical practice. Br J Psychiatry 155:754–763, 1989

Peselow ED, Stanley M, Filippi AM, et al: The predictive value of the dexamethasone suppression test. Br J Psychiatry 155:667–672, 1989

Raskind M, Eisdorfer C: The use of psychotherapeutic drugs in geriatrics, in The Use of Psychotherapeutic Drugs in the Treatment of Mental Illness. Edited by Simpson LL. New York, Raven, 1978, pp 220–244

Risse SC, Raskind MA, Nochlin D, et al: Neuropathological findings in patients with clinical diagnoses of probable Alzheimer's disease. Am J Psychiatry 147:168–172, 1990

Roffwarg H, Erman M: Evaluation and diagnosis of the sleep disorders: implications for psychiatry and other clinical specialties, in Psychiatry Update: American Psychiatric Association Annual Review, Vol 4. Edited by Hales RE, Frances AJ. Washington, DC, American Psychiatric Press, 1985, pp 294–328

Ron MA: Psychiatric manifestations of frontal lobe tumors. Br J Psychiatry 155:735–738, 1989

Sirota P, Eviatar J, Spirak B: Neurosyphilis presenting as psychiatric disorders. Br J Psychiatry 155:559–561, 1989

Snyder SH: Drug and neurotransmitter receptors in the brain. Science 224:22–28, 1985

Snyder S, Strain JJ, Wolf D: Differentiating major depression from adjustment disorder with depressed mood in the medical setting. Gen Hosp Psychiatry 12:159–165, 1990

Solomon S, Masdeu JC: Neurological evaluation, in Comprehensive Textbook of Psychiatry. Edited by Kaplan HI, Sadock BJ. Baltimore, MD, Williams & Wilkins, 1989, pp 144–176

Spitzer RL, Williams JBW, Skodol AE: DSM-III: the major achievements and an overview. Am J Psychiatry 137:151–164, 1980

Stone AA: Law, science and psychiatric malpractice: a response to Klerman's indictment of psychoanalytic psychiatry. Am J Psychiatry 147:419–427, 1990

Strayhorn JM: Control groups for psychosocial intervention outcome studies. Am J Psychiatry 144:275–282, 1987

Suddath RL, Christison GW, Torrey EF, et al: Anatomical abnormalities in the brains of monozygotic twins discordant for schizophrenia. N Engl J Med 322:789–794, 1990

Szymanski LS, Crocker AC: Mental retardation, in Comprehensive Textbook of Psychiatry. Edited by Kaplan HI, Sadock BJ. Baltimore, MD, Williams & Wilkins, 1989, pp 1728–1771

Thoren P, Asberg M, Cronholm B, et al: Clomipramine treatment of obsessive-compulsive disorder. Arch Gen Psychiatry 37:1281–1285, 1980

Watson CG, Buranen C: The frequency and identification of false positive conversion reactions. J Nerv Ment Dis 167:243–247, 1979

Waziri R: Book forum. Am J Psychiatry 147:355–356, 1990

Weinberger DR: Brain disease and psychiatric illness: when should a psychiatrist order a CAT scan? Am J Psychiatry 141:1521–1524, 1984

Whalley LJ, Christie JE, Blackwood DHR, et al: Disturbed endocrine function in the psychoses. Br J Psychiatry 155:455–461, 1989

White AJ, Barraclough B: Benefits and problems of routine laboratory investigation in adult psychiatric populations. Br J Psychiatry 155:65–72, 1989

Zohar J, Belmaker RH (eds): Treating Resistant Depression. New York, PMA Publishing, 1987

CHAPTER 4

Behavioral Formulations

UNTIL RECENTLY, BEHAVIOR THERAPY has been a stepchild of American psychiatry. Dwarfed by both psychoanalysis and biological psychiatry, behavior therapy has not been considered seriously as a viable treatment modality. For one thing, psychiatrists had relatively little formal training or experience with this perspective. For another, psychiatrists hold some assumptions about behavior therapy that are not borne out by the evidence. Marks (1986) reported that most psychiatrists believe that patients who require behavioral treatment must be referred to a behavioral specialist. Two assumptions underlie this belief. The first is that behavioral treatment requires a detailed knowledge of learning theory, and the second is that behavioral methods are too time-consuming to be useful for most busy psychiatrists. Actually, behavioral interventions can require the same or less time than is customary with psychopharmacologic treatment. That the multisite National Institute of Mental Health Treatment of Depression Collaborative Research Program (Elkins et al. 1989) chose cognitive-behavioral therapy as one of the four time-limited treatment conditions strongly suggests that behavior therapy has come of age in American psychiatry. Cognitive-behavioral therapy is a blending of traditional behavioral or conditioning methods with elements of cognitive therapy, as proposed by Beck and his colleagues (Beck 1983; Beck and Young 1985; Beck et al. 1985).

This chapter presents the behavioral formulation in the context of its theoretical premises and with regard to two formats for developing a formulation: the conditioning paradigm and the cognitive-behavioral paradigm. Finally, a behavioral formulation of the case of Mr. A followed by a step-by-step analysis of the formulation is presented.

Theoretical Premises of Behavior Therapy

Grounded in experimental psychological research, behavior therapy is derived from the concepts and principles of learning theory as developed by behavioral psychiatrists such as Joseph Wolpe, Isaac Marks, and Steward Agras and by the cognitive-oriented psychiatrists such as Aaron Beck, David Burns, and John Rush. Actually, *behavior therapy* is an umbrella term for a wide variety of distinct groups or approaches. At one end of a continuum are Skinner, Lewinsohn, Wolpe, and Eysenck, representing objective behaviorism. For them, only what can be described as measurable and observable behaviors are deemed relevant for treatment and change. At the other end of the continuum are Beck, Mowrer, Meichenbaum, and Schwartz, representing cognitive behaviorism. For this group, cognitions and mental imagery are also considered important in the assessment and treatment of patients. Between these endpoints are a number of distinct behavior therapies, such as covert conditioning, self-instructional training, problem-solving therapy, self-control therapy, personal science, and rational behavior therapy (Kendall and Bacon 1988).

There is a wide range of opinion about what constitutes behavior therapy. Four general premises about the behavioral approach that would be endorsed by the majority of behaviorists are

1. A patient's problems are understood, in part, as disordered thoughts, feelings, or behavior causally related to antecedent events.
2. A patient's problems are understood, in part, as disordered thoughts, feelings, or behavior resulting from reinforcing consequences of behavior.
3. A patient's problems are understood, in part, as a result of dysfunctional cognition or behavioral deficits.
4. A patient's condition is known to be treatable, in part, by specific cognitive or behavioral techniques.

The Conditioning Paradigm

In the conditioning paradigm, maladaptive behavior results from either a deficiency of functional learning or an acquisition of dysfunctional learning. Maladaptive behavior is not viewed as a superficial "symptom" or manifestation of an underlying disease process or disorder, nor is it considered a substitute for a conflict or the unconscious expression of a blocked desire. Rather, it is a learned response that has detrimental consequences for the patient and the patient's environment, regardless of how it was acquired. Behavioral analysis is the sine qua non of this paradigm. It provides guidelines for assessing the nature, severity, and frequency of the specified behavior and its functional relationship with environmental antecedents and consequences. It is assumed that a patient is best understood and described by what he or she does in a particular situation. These maladaptive behaviors can be treated through the systematic application of empirically derived behavioral procedures. Treatment is directed either toward reducing or eliminating the intensity or frequency of the maladaptive behavior or learning more adaptive behavior. Interventions are focused on rendering improvement in measurable, specific behavior. Treatment is based on a careful analysis of the problem into components and is targeted specifically and systematically (Glynn et al. 1989). Earlier proponents of this paradigm adopted a clinician-centered approach to treatment. Recently, this view has begun to change, and patient involvement in the treatment process is sought.

The Cognitive-Behavioral Paradigm

Under the rubric of cognitive-behavioral therapy are such diverse approaches as cognitive therapy, rational-emotive therapy, self-instructional training, coping-skills therapy, problem-solving therapy, and self-inoculation training. Although there are some conceptual differences, it is possible to specify the premises that characterize what most cognitive behaviorists believe.

The basic starting point is that persons respond primarily to cognitive representation of their environment rather than to the environment per se. Most human learning is cognitively mediated. Thoughts, feelings, and behaviors are causally interrelated, and attitudes, expectations, and attributions are central to producing, predicting, and understanding abnormal behavior. It is also believed that cognitive processes can be cast into testable formulations that are easily integrated with the conditioning paradigm, and it is possible and desirable to combine cognitive treatment strategies with enactive techniques and conditioning methods. The clinician is a diagnostician, educator, and technical consultant whose tasks are to assess maladaptive cognitive processes and collaborate with the patient to design learning experiences that may mediate these dysfunctional cognitions and the behavior and mood states with which they correlate (Kendall and Bacon 1988). Treatment strategies are individually tailored to different problems in different individuals.

In this paradigm, interventions tend to be active, time limited, and fairly structured. Therapy is designed to help the patient identify, reality test, and correct maladaptive or dysfunctional cognitions. The patient is aided in recognizing connections among cognitions, moods, and behaviors as well as their consequences. The patient is encouraged to become aware of and monitor the role of negative thoughts and images and to challenge and change them. Treatment continues beyond the scope of the session through the use of homework assignments, such that the patient eventually learns to become his or her own therapist. Ultimately, self-management is the goal of this approach.

Finally, it should be noted that cognitive-behavioral therapists also use environmental manipulations, but they do so for different reasons than conditioning therapists. For the cognitive-behavioral therapist, such manipulations represent informational feedback trials that provide the patient an opportunity to question, reappraise, and acquire self-control over maladaptive cognitions, moods, and behaviors (Meichenbaum and Turk 1983).

Paradigms in Behavior Therapy: Past, Present, and Future

In this section, we briefly review the dominant paradigms of behavior therapy over the past 40 years as well as anticipate the most likely paradigms in the near future.

As behavior therapy developed in the 1950s and 1960s, the conditioning model was its paradigm. The conditioning paradigm embodied two subclasses: classical conditioning and operant conditioning. Both of these subclasses rigorously held to the tenets of the same objectivist and logical positivist stance that informed the early biological paradigm.

Logical positivism assumes that there is an external world independent of human experience. Objective knowledge about this world can be obtained only through direct sensory experience. In this view, observations are the ultimate truths on which scientists can achieve agreement because observations are objective. A statement that succinctly captures the essence of this epistemology is, If it exists it can be measured, and if it can be measured it exists. This view is similar to the disease perspective of McHugh and Slavney (1983).

The 1970s and 1980s witnessed the "cognitive revolution" and the shift from the conditioning-only paradigm to the cognitive-behavioral paradigm. Kendall and Bacon (1988) viewed the change as more of a "paradigm drift" than a full "paradigm shift." They argued that cumulative changes arose among various individual researchers and clinicians in response to the limitations of the conditioning paradigm to account for cognitively mediated conceptions of behavior. These authors also noted that the change in paradigms was greatly influenced by the pervasive computer and cognitive information processing phenomenon experienced throughout the world in the last 15 years. Woolfork (1988) suggested that fundamental changes in assumptions about human nature and the human condition also influence the shift to the cognitive-behavioral paradigm.

A number of cognitive behaviorists argue that the logical positivist view of science is flawed and must be replaced by a social constructivist view, in which reality is seen as a social reaction or construction rather than an externally discoverable or observable entity. The cognitive-behavioral perspective embodies features that are the constructivist view (Erwin 1988). From the idiographic perspective, data about the patient as a unique individual are often more useful than objective data. This constructivist perspective is similar to the life-story perspective of McHugh and Slavney (1983).

Fishman et al. (1988) polled 10 prominent behavioral therapists as to their perception of the dominant paradigm and epistemology in the field of behavior therapy today. They unanimously agreed that the dominant paradigm was the cognitive behavioral, although the dominant epistemology was still objectivistic. When asked to predict the trends for behavior therapy in the future, there was marked disagreement. More than half believed that constructivism would become the dominant epistemology. But there was considerable disparity about the dominant paradigm, which ranged from a return to the conditioning paradigm to an existential-phenomenological version of cognitive-behavioral therapy.

Format for Developing a Behavioral Conditioning Formulation

In the conditioning paradigm, a formulation is described as a hypothesis that 1) relates all of the presenting complaints to one another, 2) explains why these difficulties have developed, and 3) provides predictions of the patient's behavior given any stimulus conditions (Wolpe and Turkat 1985). Such a formulation is based on a complete behavioral analysis. This behavioral analysis is accomplished, in large part, during the course of a behavioral interview. Information is elicited in a logical and systematic way. Hypothesis testing is the basic interview strategy. The clinician must quickly develop hypotheses and then test them until they have been accepted or rejected. If the clinician is unsure as to what information to seek, it is unlikely that the patient will get the type of treatment he or she requires.

Relating to the Patient

The way the clinician relates to the patient is critical in formulation and treatment. The behavior therapist must be able to empathize with the patient. However, the form this empathy takes is different from that of the psychoanalyst or Rogerian. For the behaviorist, empathy is demonstrated when the clinician can accurately predict the patient's behavior. Wolpe and Turkat (1985) noted that an effective therapeutic relationship exists when the clinician has created an environment for the patient that enables the clinician to get the information needed to make accurate predictions.

Guidelines for Developing a Formulation

To the extent that the conditioning paradigm takes a collaborative focus, the stops by which information is elicited will vary in sequence from case to casc. Nevertheless, Wolpe and Turkat (1985) indicated some general guidelines: 1) the specification of all of the patient's problems, 2) the onset or precipitant of each problem, 3) the development and maintenance of each problem, and 4) the etiologic and predisposing factors. The etiology of the problematic behavior provides the core for developing the conditioning formulation and treatment plan. Essentially, the behavioral interview is an etiologic inquiry that addresses predisposing factors, traces the problem from its onset to present development, and establishes the conditions that maintain or perpetuate it.

Step 1: Specifying the problems. From the first interview, the clinician must attend to the patient in all spheres by surveying dress, posture and motions, eye patterns, breathing patterns, skin color, and so on. The clinician is searching for any clues about the patient. A typical general opening questions is, "What seems to be the problem?" Depending on the patient's response, the clinician focuses on the presenting complaint and its perpetuating or maintaining factors, before proceeding to the specification of other problems. There is no standard order of questioning. Hypotheses and data determine the flow and sequencing of the interview.

Because the behavioral formulation is based on specific hypotheses, the clinician seeks to generate an initial hypothesis as soon as possible in the first interview. While observing the patient's nonverbal behavior and style and listening to the presenting problem, the clinician begins to generate hypotheses, gather data, and test hypotheses. As much as possible, the clinician tries to understand exactly what the patient means, for example, by the word *depression.* Parameters of each response are specified, including intensity, duration, frequency, and sequencing with other responses.

Step 2: Specifying the onset or precipitant of each problem. Following the specification of each problem, the clinician's inquiry can follow either of two lines. The clinician may examine the onset of the problem or investigate its maintaining factors. Specifying the onset or precipitant is briefly discussed here. Precipitants refer to antecedent conditions that trigger or coincide with the onset of symptoms or maladaptive behaviors. Strict attention is paid to environmental factors that were present at the onset and first manifestation of the problem: where it was, what time of day, who was there, what was said and done, what happened next, and so on. An exhaustive specification of the independent and dependent variables should clarify the onset of each problem. The precise antecedents and their effects on behavior are delineated. The response systems affected and their manifestations (e.g., elevated heart rate, lightheadedness) are operationalized as well.

Step 3: Specifying the perpetuating factors. Perpetuating or maintaining refers to consequences that reinforce and continue a given behavior. These consequences are usually psychological or social, but they may also be physical (e.g., habituation to an addictive substance). Hypothesized perpetuating factors are established by precise delineation of antecedents and consequences.

Step 4: Specifying the predisposing and etiologic factors. Once the onset and the development and maintaining information are derived, a search for predisposing factors is begun. The clinician's task is to identify those environmental and genetic factors that promoted the patient's susceptibility or vulnerability to develop the current problem given certain circumstances and conditions.

Wolpe (1982) identified several factors that have common predisposing conditions for a number of psychiatric disorders. These included early family experiences, parental and sibling characteristics, interaction styles, religious training, educational experience, social relations, and sexual experiences. For example, the shy and avoidant patient is likely to have parental models for such behavior (i.e., vicarious learning) that favored a lack of opportunities to acquire appropriate interpersonal behaviors and social skills (i.e., operant conditioning). The patient may have also been involved in traumatic events and consequences, such as rejection by peers, resulting in the present avoidant personality pattern and social anxiety (i.e., classical conditioning).

Specifying and Presenting the Formulation

The behavioral conditioning formulation developed by the clinician is typically written in a formal report, although it may also be verbally presented to the patient. In its written form, the formulation can be laid out in five sections: 1) a description of the presenting problems, 2) the history and the onset or precipitants, 3) the maintaining or perpetuating factors, 4) the etiologic and predisposing variables, and 5) the behavioral treatment plan based on the first four sections.

Behavior therapists like Wolpe and Turkat (1985) emphasized the value of verbally presenting the formulation to the patient. Besides increasing the patient's understanding of the findings, formulation, and treatment focus, the patient is socialized in thc conditioning paradigm and its theory and language. Because the patient is invited to comment on, evaluate, and confirm or refute all aspects of the formulation, the patient is more likely to become engaged in the collaborative process of treatment. This discussion also has the effect of solidifying the clinician's confidence in it.

Wolpe and Turkat (1985) suggested that the clinician begin the presentation with a statement such as, "Given the information you have provided me, I would like to give you my view of what the problems are, and why they developed." The clinician then describes the presenting problem and discusses the predisposing, precipitating, and perpetuating conditions. The patient's unique history is interwoven so that the patient can understand and then comment on the clinician's formulation. Since the presentation of the formulation has been preceded by earlier shaping of the patient's conceptualization of the problems and their development, the patient has been "shaped" toward the clinician's understanding, and the formal presentation serves to tie all the data together.

Format for Developing a Cognitive-Behavioral Paradigm

In the cognitive-behavioral paradigm, a formulation is a hypothesis about underlying deficits producing the patient's problems. The formulation serves as the clinician's compass, guiding treatment planning and intervention. More specifically, a well-articulated cognitive-behavioral formulation can guide the choice of treatment, modality, intervention strategy, and point of intervention as well as predict and manage noncompliance (Persons 1989).

The cognitive-behavioral formulation strategy and format developed by Persons (1989) consists of six steps:

1. Specify a problem list.
2. Propose the underlying mechanism.
3. Relate the mechanism to the specified problems.
4. Indicate the precipitant(s) of the specified problems.
5. Specify the early life origins of the patient's central problems/mechanism.
6. Predict obstacles to treatment based on the formulation.

Step 1: Specify a Problem List

The first step is to specify the patient's problem list. The problem list should be all-inclusive. Typically, a patient's list may contain 8–10 items. These might include depression, insomnia, panic attacks, eating problems, procrastination, drug and alcohol abuse, phobias, obsessive thoughts, rituals, memory problems, marital conflicts, social isolation, unemployment, housing problems, financial difficulties, headaches, and other medical problems. Even though the patient may resist providing a comprehensive listing of concerns, the clinician cannot hope to formulate the case accurately or to intervene successfully without an inclusive list. Because of unawareness, embarrassment, or unwillingness to change certain behaviors, a patient may initially withhold some problem areas. An explanation of the importance of disclosure and a comprehensive assessment can aid the specification of the problem list. Quantitative measures such as rating scales or activity logs can be used to assess a variety of behavioral aspects of problems.

Problems can be specified at both "macro" and "micro" levels. At the macro level, overt difficulties include depression, insomnia, and obesity. These are often the presenting problems noted by patients. At the micro level, problems can be specified in terms of three components: cognitions, behaviors, and moods. At this level of specification, the nature of the problem and its underlying mechanism become clearer.

A cognitive component can be isolated for basically all problems, including those that do not at first appear to involve cognitions. Negative mood states, images, and automatic thoughts are associated with most behaviors. For instance, when a secretary jammed a copying machine, she experienced fear and a barrage of cognitive processes, including, "I never do anything right," and the image of her boss firing her on the spot.

A behavioral component may include overt motor behavior, physiologic sequences, and verbalizations. Identifying manifestations of this component is particularly necessary for cognitive-behavioral formulations. Discovering that the patient spends daytime hours in bed watching television, overeating, yelling obscenities at his wife, or experiencing palpitations and dizziness is useful information.

A mood component is also elicited. Mood is the patient's subjective report of the patient's emotional experiences, which are typically negative and unpleasant. Common moods are depression, anxiety, anger, frustration, jealousy, and hopelessness. Like the behavioral and cognitive components, moods are useful in understanding and clarifying the patient's problems.

All three micro components—cognitive, behavioral, and mood—tend to reflect the maladaptive underlying mechanism. For example, a homemaker presenting with panic attacks (problem) is experiencing intense fear and anxiety (behaviors) and self-talk such as, "I'm trapped, I'm going to die" (cognition).

Step 2: Propose the Underlying Mechanism

The underlying mechanism is the heart of the cognitive-behavioral formulation. The basic tenet of the cognitive-behavioral paradigm is that an underlying central problem produces the overt difficulty. After specifying the problem list, the clinician proposes a single explanation—a problem or deficit—that is responsible for producing the patient's overt difficulties. This explanation must be broad enough to account for all of the problems on the list. This explanatory mechanism can usually be stated as a central irrational belief such as, "If I get too close to people, I'll get hurt" or "If I don't do everything perfectly, I'll be rejected." These central beliefs are usually framed in an if-then format, such as, "If I'm very successful, then others will accept me." But occasionally they are simpler, blanket statements, such as, "I'm a worthless bum" or "No one loves me." There is considerable theorizing about the types of central mechanisms underlying depressive disorders, anxiety disorders, and severe personality disorders, but to date only a paucity of research data support these theories.

For depressive disorders, Seligman's (1975) "learned helplessness" hypothesis has been widely discussed. In learned helplessness, the individual fails to see that his or her responses can affect the outcome of a particular predicament. Helplessness is first learned through experiencing an inescapable situation that produces, through a mediating cognition, a failure to connect the aversive stimulus with an escape response.

Beck (1983) and others described two types of dysfunctional beliefs that underlie depressive symptoms: those involving autonomy and those involving overdependency. Depressed individuals with problems of autonomy believe they must be highly accomplished, achieving, and independent to be worthwhile. Depressed individuals with problems of dependency believe they must be liked, loved, or approved of by others to be worthwhile.

Regarding the anxiety disorders, Beck et al. (1985) proposed that anxious individuals believe themselves to be vulnerable to danger and unable to cope. When faced with difficult circumstances, these individuals are likely to respond with anxiety syndromes. Cognitive therapists have recently begun to focus on the personality disorders. Young (unpublished manuscript) elaborated various maladaptive schemata that underlie personality disorders. He described 15 schemata that cluster into four groups: autonomy, connectedness, worthiness, and limits and standards. Smucker (1990) suggested that three early maladaptive schemata are common in the patient with borderline personality disorder. These borderline schemata are 1) abandonment, the belief that people I get close to will leave me; 2) mistrust, the belief that I can't trust others; and 3) dependency, the belief that I need others to take care of me because I can't do it alone.

Persons (1989) noted that the process of developing a hypothesis about the underlying mechanism is one of the most difficult and challenging aspects of the cognitive-behavioral approach. She suggested that the clinician begin by examining the problem list and by asking the question, "What do all these problems have in common?" The steps in developing the underlying mechanism are 1) examine the problem list, 2) study the chief complaint, 3) examine the automatic thoughts, and 4) look for antecedents and consequences.

Step 3: Relate the Underlying Mechanism to the Problems

At this step, the clinician works to specify the way in which the hypothesized central dysfunction problem produces the problems on the list. For example, a middle-aged business executive presenting with depression, relationship difficulties, excessive procrastination on the job, and sexual impotence may have the central dysfunction belief: "Unless I do things perfectly, I will be rejected." Here, problems of job, interpersonal relations, and sexual performance can be understood as resulting from his fear of failure to perform perfectly and the resulting rejection. Similarly, his depressive symptoms can be understood as an indirect result of the lack of gratification or satisfaction he experiences in his life, along with his intense self-criticism due to his perceived failures and personal inadequacies.

Step 4: Indicate Precipitants of Current Problems

Specifying precipitants of current problems is the next step. The more a precipitant reflects the central mechanism, the more the proposed central mechanism is confirmed. For example, it could be predicted that the perfectionist businessman noted above would become depressed after failure to meet an important deadline that his boss had set for him.

Step 5: Specify the Origins of the Central Problem

Then the clinician attempts to chronicle the possible origins of the central problem or mechanism in the patient's early life history. Relationships with parents usually play a central role. For instance, the perfectionist businessman gave a history of being reared by parents who held extraordinarily high expectations for achievement and also criticized him for even the smallest errors or infractions. He learned to do things perfectly because making mistakes led to criticism and rejection.

Step 6: Predict Obstacles to Treatment

Finally, the clinician anticipates a course of treatment and how the patient is likely to engage in and participate in treatment. By anticipating obstacles and difficulties that may arise, the clinician is more likely to prevent or solve them. For example, a clinician working with the perfectionist businessman might anticipate that the patient will procrastinate with intersession assignments or that he may be overly sensitive to clarifications and interpretations that he perceives are critical.

This six-part format can serve as the outline for the written formulation. The clinician is encouraged to write at least one or more sentences for each of the six steps.

Like Wolpe and Turkat (1985), Persons (1989) also suggested that the formulation should be discussed with the patient. If the patient believes that the formulation is accurate, the clinician has supporting evidence for it. If the patient believes the formulation is not accurate, the clinician needs to consider other possible explanations or underlying mechanisms.

Behavioral Formulation of the Case of Mr. A

A behavioral formulation of the case of Mr. A follows. Note that separate conditioning and cognitive-behavioral etiologic formulation statements are included, as well as a treatment plan encompassing both paradigms.

Summary Statement

At the age of 42, Mr. A is experiencing his first episode of major depression. There is probable evidence for a DSM-III-R (American Psychiatric Association 1987) diagnosis of obsessive-compulsive personality disorder.

Problems, Onset, and Maintaining Factors

Mr. A has experienced a profound change in his behavior over a 6-week period. Most obvious are the vegetative symptoms associated with clinical depression: insomnia, anhedonia, weight loss, and recurrent thoughts of death. In addition to depressive features, a number of other problems, some of much longer duration, are noted. These include limited closeness, marital discord, possible sexual dysfunction, limited social relating skills, and an obsessive-perfectionist style. Mr. A overprioritizes his career at the expense of family and personal needs. This is expressed as "workaholism" and limited leisure interests and pursuits. Notable are the limited number of response-contingent reinforcers in his environment (i.e., the relatively few pleasant stimuli available even before depressive symptoms were expressed). The most likely precipitant for the depressive episode is his failure to be promoted. The loss of a source of personal reinforcement due to the ongoing sexual and emotional withdrawal by his wife and perhaps even the endings of an unreported extramarital affair may be additional precipitants. Factors that serve as perpetuants or maintaining factors for Mr. A's workaholism, perfectionism, limited leisure activities, and limited support network of friends are likely to be response contingencies associated with his job, such as his boss's and co-workers' recognition of his hard work, productivity, long hours, and dedication. It is unlikely that he has received much positive reinforcement from his family, particularly his wife. This suggests that his career is his principal source of reinforcement, and the reduction, loss, or threat of this reinforcement will greatly affect him.

Two Formulations

Conditioning formulation. Being passed over for promotion and having a limited number of response-contingent reinforcers have probably resulted in Mr. A's depressive features. Furthermore, Mr. A appears to be predisposed to depression, given his hard-working, hyperresponsible, and self-sacrificing style. This style may have been modeled from Mr. A's mother, a single parent who was probably often absent physically and emotionally when he was a child. As a hyperresponsible oldest child, Mr. A likely received little nurturing. He had little time or opportunity to learn the kind of social relating skills and leisure interests and pursuits that would have provided an important source of support and pleasure as he coped with his current losses and disappointments. He was positively reinforced for his achievement and attention to detail and probably punished for leisure (i.e., nonachievement). This predisposition and genetic loading and male modeling of depression, desertion, and suicide suggest that Mr. A's thoughts about death need to be carefully evaluated despite his denial of suicidal ideation.

Cognitive-behavioral formulation. Being passed over for promotion and the loss of personal reinforcements appear to have activated a number of underlying assumptions and negative schemata, resulting in Mr. A's depressive features. Mr. A probably views his worth as dependent on being highly productive and successful while avoiding mistakes and the disapproval of others at all costs. He works diligently and compulsively, accounting for his perfectionist, self-sacrificing style and his need to be in control. This single-mindedness leaves little room for leisure pursuits, satisfying relationships, or emotional expression of his needs. As a child, Mr. A probably learned to construct reality in accord with negative schemata involving themes of defectiveness, failure, and subjugation. Accordingly, he adopted the belief that he was basically inadequate, defective, and unlovable and must sacrifice and subjugate his needs in favor of others. As these negative schemata are activated, Mr. A will likely distort events in a way that maintains these assumptions and schemes. He will view himself as a failure, the environment as overwhelming and unsupportive, and the future as hopeless. Because a sense of hopelessness correlates highly with completed suicide, his suicide potential should be carefully evaluated. Mr. A's limited sources of positive reinforcement and social support are likely to exacerbate, confirm, and reinforce his sense of failure and loss.

Treatment Plan

Conditioning component. Because of his reduced number of response-contingent reinforcers, a major component of Mr. A's treatment will involve increasing the number of his pleasant experiences. The clinician will collaborate with Mr. A to devise a personalized list of pleasant events and attempt to increase their number. This might be accomplished with a homework assignment to complete a certain number of pleasant events on a daily basis. The clinician will work with Mr. A to overcome obstacles to this task. Selected social skills training will be initiated to improve both the quality and quantity of social interactions. Relaxation training and distraction procedures will be undertaken to help secure restful sleep and diminish nocturnal ruminations. In addition, an exercise regimen with daily quotas will be instituted.

Cognitive-behavioral component. The mainstay of treatment involves cognitive strategies for recognizing and diminishing negative assumptions and schemata involving perfectionism, defectiveness, failure, and subjugation and to develop or increase positive attributions and interactions. The central theme to treatment planning will be to help Mr. A revise and restructure his assumptions and schemata. Homework assignments will be made to reinforce these activities.

The marital situation will be explored further, and, if appropriate, couples therapy will be suggested to modify interactions in which Mr. A's wife may be reinforcing his helplessness. The therapy may also need to address any treatable sexual dysfunction disorder.

In view of the biological features of Mr. A's illness, treatment with medication will be suggested, but acceptance will depend on his attributions and beliefs about the appropriateness of medication and its possible efficacy. Mr. A's high need for control might well create a reluctance to take drugs. If initiated, however, adherence will probably be excellent. Concurrent drug and behavioral treatment can be synergistic and beneficial.

By the end of the first treatment session, the therapist will ensure that Mr. A understands the nature and rationale of behavior therapy and be prepared to deal with fluctuations in mood during treatment. Target symptoms will have been selected, and specific goals set. Subsequent therapy will be interactive and verbal. Interpretations will be avoided, although from time to time Mr. A might be invited to speculate about behaviors or cognitions. Each session will be carefully planned, an agenda will be agreed on with Mr. A, and his feedback will be frequently elicited to ensure mutual understanding and collaboration.

The immediate prognosis is excellent, based on the fact that this is a first episode in an individual with high levels of achievement. Mr. A's personality style will be conducive to strong collaboration in therapy based on a need for mastery. The prognosis for the marriage is less certain, based on the wife's possible preference for her husband in his depressed state.

Step-by-Step Analysis of the Case Formulation

The purpose of this section is to provide the reader with a sense of how the preceding case formulation was conceptualized and written. Accordingly, each of the components of the formulation will be discussed, except for the summary statement, which needs no comment.

Problems, Onset, and Maintaining Factors

Two different formats were proposed to help the clinician conceptualize the behavioral formulation process. Although there are considerable differences between the conditioning format of Wolpe and Turkat (1985) and the cognitive-behavioral format of Persons (1989) regarding etiology/underlying mechanism, there is considerable similarity on the other dimensions. Wolpe and Turkat's format calls for specification of problems, onset, maintaining factors, and predisposing factors. Persons's format suggests similar terms: problem list, precipitant, relation of mechanism to problems, and origins of the central problems. Because of these similarities, comments on this component are essentially the same for both formats.

Ten specific problems were listed besides the most obvious presenting concern: depression and its neurovegetative features. The authors of both formats require that a number of problems or problem areas be listed, in addition to the presenting concern.

But how was this list of 10 problems generated from the case material on Mr. A? A careful reading of the case suggested a number of areas of functioning that needed to be examined: work, relations with his wife and children, social relations, and leisure activities. For each of these areas, the clinician attempts to isolate instances of dysfunctional behavior, cognitions, or moods. Often this is aided by a knowledge of clinical syndromes and their associated clusters of behavior. For instance, depressed individuals typically show decreased activity at work, at home, and in social and intimate relations. This certainly was true of Mr. A. In addition to such short-term problems, there are difficulties that are more long term and usually characterological in nature. For Mr. A, these are represented by his compulsive and perfectionist style—suggested by the Axis II diagnosis of obsessive-compulsive personality disorder.

Specifying the onset or precipitant(s) was made easy because the case material suggested a failure to be promoted as the immediate precipitant.

The clinician might also look beyond the given information and wonder if other potential losses or failed expectations may have been additional precipitants. For instance, had Mr. A been engaged in an extramarital relationship that had recently terminated, or had he lost a large sum of money in an investment around the time the promotion was announced?

From a behavioral perspective, antecedent, behavior, and consequence (A-B-C) is central to a behavioral analysis. From the case material, we note the impact of an antecedent event, such as failure to be promoted, on Mr. A's behavior. The consequences or reinforcers that have sustained Mr. A's hard-working, self-sacrificing, and perfectionist features need to be considered, because when these positive reinforcers are reduced or replaced with aversive stimuli, we expect Mr. A's behavior to change.

Conceptualizing the Formulation Statements

Wolpe and Turkat (1985) used the term *etiology*, Persons (1989) used the term *underlying mechanism*, to describe why a patient is symptomatic and dysfunctional. To describe both the conditioning and cognitive-behavioral formulations, it is necessary to review some theory about depression for both paradigms.

A highly regarded explanation of depression in the conditioning paradigm was advanced by Lewinsohn et al. (1984, 1986), who believe that a depressed patient suffers from a reduced number of response-contingent reinforcers. The patient experiences few, if any, pleasant events. As a result, the patient's rate of responding is reduced, and the patient experiences symptoms of depression. Lewinsohn et al. also indicated that the patient who is predisposed to clinical depression is deficient in social skills and subsequently receives even lower levels of social reinforcement. They proposed that depression results from a reduction of antecedent evolving events in a patient with limited social skills and social supports. The patient then experiences disrupted automatic or scripted patterns, leading to decreased response-contingent reinforcers. This results in the emotional, behavioral, and interpersonal correlates of depression. If this becomes continuous, the patient becomes more symptomatic and experiences increased self-criticism, social withdrawal, and intensification of negative affect. This "vicious cycle" serves to maintain the depressed state.

The cognitive-behavioral theory of depression developed by Beck (1983) and refined and articulated by Beck and Young (1985) was the formulation for the cognitive-behavioral basis of the case of Mr. A. According to Beck and Young, negative cognition is the core process in depression and is reflected in the cognitive triad of depression. The triad consists of negative beliefs the patient holds about the self, the world or environment, and the future. This triad reflects the patient's automatic thoughts, underlying assumptions, and negative schemata. The most important predisposing factor for depression is the presence of early negative schemata. Beck and Young maintained that the child learns to construct reality through his or her early experiences with the environment, particularly with significant others. These schemata tend to be outside one's awareness and dormant until a life event, such as Mr. A's failure to be promoted, activates the schemata. Once activated, the schemata predispose the patient to distort events in a predictable and characteristic fashion. This will then be reflected in the cognitive triad and the symptoms of depression.

With respect to Lewinsohn et al.'s (1984, 1986) theory of depression, there are a number of points of "fit" between the case data and the theory. Mr. A is deficient in a number of social skills and a support system. For instance, he is probably a proper, fairly rigid, no-nonsense kind of person who is out of touch with his own feelings and probably remains emotionally distant from others. What few friends he has are probably co-workers. It is unlikely that he shares his personal concerns with any of them. It is questionable whether he is even comfortable self-disclosing with his wife. He seems to have so narrowly defined his world that he gets little if any reinforcement or support outside of his job. Because his expectation of being promoted has failed, and he has lost interest in his work, his response-contingent reinforcers now appear to be minimal if not nearly absent. Because of his social skills deficits, Mr. A is predisposed for clinical depression. This predisposition probably results from both operant conditioning and modeling. Because he was the oldest sibling, Mr. A was required to help raise the others and hold a job at an early age. The histories of hyperresponsible children like Mr. A suggest that they received little nurturing from their caregivers. They are reinforced for their hard work and self-sacrifice. This was probably the behavior modeled from Mr. A's mother. We could predict, therefore, that Mr. A would present with depressive features after being passed over for a job promotion.

With respect to Beck's (1983) theory of depression, data about Mr. A also "fit" well with the theory. A common theme among the items on the problem list is perfectionism. The underlying assumption about perfectionism, "My worth depends on being successful while avoiding mistakes," is derived from the case material and inferred from his Axis II diagnosis of obsessive-compulsive personality disorder. Young (unpublished manuscript) listed some 15 negative schemata. Of these, Mr. A has probably internalized 3. The defectiveness-unlovability schema involves the feeling that one is unworthy, defective, or fundamentally unlovable to significant others. The failure-competence schema embodies the belief that one cannot perform competently in areas of career, responsibilities to self or others, or decision making. The subjugation–lack of individuation schema involves the voluntary or involuntary surrender of one's own needs to satisfy others' needs with an accompanying failure to recognize one's own needs. These schemata appear to have been activated by the failed expectation(s) of Mr. A. Besides being passed over for promotion, other losses may have contributed to the activation of these schemata and hence to Mr. A's clinical depression.

Treatment Plan

The initial suggestion to work on increasing pleasant events is supported by several empirical studies (Blaney 1977; Persons 1989) and is basic to Lewinsohn et al.'s (1984, 1986) approach to the treatment of depression. Furthermore, Lewinsohn and associates recommended relaxation and social skills training (1984) and suggested how the clinician can utilize bibliotherapy (1986) or a time-limited group to accomplish these. Note that the first paragraph of the treatment plan section focuses exclusively on the amelioration of depressive symptoms and short-term problems.

A general strategy in the behavioral paradigms is to target specific intervention for each of the problems on the problem list, focusing first on the short-term problem. If the patient is willing to continue in treatment, the longer-term relational and characterological problems are then addressed. For such problems as Mr. A's perfectionist style and dysfunctional life priorities, cognitive restructuring would be the treatment of choice. Couples therapy would likely involve operant conditioning, psychoeducation, and cognitive restructuring interventions. Behavior and cognitive-behavioral therapists emphasize the value of enhancing treatment compliance or adherence. These therapists work to reduce resistance and relapse by establishing a collaborative relationship with the patient (Meichenbaum and Turk 1983). Because research and clinical experience also show that medication in combination with behavioral and cognitive-behavioral interventions can act synergistically (Elkins et al. 1989), an antidepressant was considered. Moreover, mention is made of the patient's potential difficulties in responding to treatment based on his Axis II feature. Finally, a statement about the patient's overall prognosis rounds out the treatment point of the formulation.

References

American Psychiatric Association: Diagnostic and Statistical Manual of Mental Disorders, 3rd Edition, Revised. Washington, DC, American Psychiatric Association, 1987

Beck AT: Cognitive therapy of depression: new perspectives, in Treatment of Depression: Old Controversies and New Approaches. Edited by Clayton PJ, Barrett JE. New York, Raven, 1983, pp 213–232

Beck AT, Young JE: Depression, in Clinical Handbook of Psychological Disorders. Edited by Barlow DH. New York, Guilford, 1985, pp 206–244

Beck AT, Emery G, Greenberg BL: Anxiety Disorders and Phobias: A Cognitive Perspective. New York, Basic Books, 1985

Blaney PH: Contemporary theories of depression: critique and comparison. J Abnorm Psychol 86:203–223, 1977

Elkins I, Shea T, Watkins JT, et al: National Institute of Mental Health Treatment of Depression Collaborative Research Program. Arch Gen Psychiatry 46:971–982, 1989

Erwin E: Cognitivist and behaviorist paradigms in clinical psychology, in Paradigms in Behavior Therapy: Present and Promise. Edited by Fishman DB, Rotgers F, Franks CM. New York, Springer, 1988, pp 109–140

Fishman DB, Rotgers F, Franks CM: Paradigmatic decision making in behavior therapy: a provisional roadmap, in Paradigms in Behavior Therapy: Present and Promise. Edited by Fishman DB, Rotgers F, Franks CM. New York, Springer, 1988, pp 323–362

Glynn SM, Meuser CT, Liberman RP: The behavioral approach, in Outpatient Psychiatry: Diagnosis and Treatment, 2nd Edition. Edited by Lazare A. Baltimore, MD, Williams & Wilkins, 1989, pp 59–68

Kendall PC, Bacon SF: Cognitive behavior therapy, in Paradigms in Behavior Therapy: Present and Promise, Edited by Fishman DB, Rotgers F, Franks CM. New York, Springer, 1988, pp 141–167

Lewinsohn PM, Steinmetz J, Autonuccio DO, et al: The Coping With Depression Course: A Psychoeducational Intervention for Unipolar Depression. Eugene, OR, Castalia Publishing, 1984

Lewinsohn PM, Munoz RF, Youngren MA, et al: Control Your Depression. Englewood Cliffs, NJ, Prentice-Hall, 1986

Marks I: Behavioral psychotherapy in general psychiatry helping patients to help themselves. Br J Psychiatry 150:593–597, 1986

McHugh PR, Slavney PR: The Perspectives of Psychiatry. Baltimore, MD, Johns Hopkins University Press, 1983

Meichenbaum D, Turk D: Pain and Behavioral Medicine: A Cognitive Behavioral Approach. New York, Guilford, 1983

Persons JB: Cognitive Therapy in Practice: A Case Formulation Approach. New York, WW Norton, 1989

Seligman ME: Helplessness: On Depression, Death and Development. San Francisco, CA, WH Freeman, 1975

Smucker M: Cognitive therapy lecture series. Milwaukee, Medical College of Wisconsin, February 26, 1990

Wolpe J: The Practice of Behavior Therapy, 3rd Edition. Elmsford, NY, Pergamon, 1982

Wolpe J, Turkat ID: Behavioral formulations of clinical cases, in Behavioral Case Formulation. Edited by Turkat ID. New York, Plenum, 1985, pp 5–36

Woolfork RL: The self in cognitive behavior therapy, in Paradigms in Behavior Therapy: Present and Promise. Edited by Fishman DB, Rotgers F, Franks CM. New York, Springer, 1988, pp 168–184

CHAPTER 5

Biopsychosocial Formulations

FEW WOULD QUESTION THAT PSYCHIATRY has undergone a significant paradigm shift away from psychoanalysis during the last three decades (Abrams 1981; Cummings 1990). This transformation has been due to many factors, some obvious and others more subtle. Of primary importance has been the desire by many psychiatrists to have a method of integrating diverse clinical material about patients in a balanced way that is helpful in designing effective treatment strategies (Kline and Cameron 1978; Strauss 1975). The virtual explosion of well-documented data pertaining to the importance of biological, psychological, behavioral, and sociocultural factors in psychiatric diseases and their treatments has made a rigid, reductionistic adherence to one theoretical point of view untenable (Fink 1988; Goldsmith and Mandell 1969; Lazare 1989). Changing political and economic realities of psychiatric practice have forced psychiatrists to consider combinations of treatment methods that are not only effective but also cost efficient (Sharfstein and Beigel 1985; Sperry 1988). Engel's (1980) biopsychosocial model and other eclectic, pluralistic, and multidimensional modifications of it (Abrams 1981, 1983; Cleghorn 1985; Lazare 1989; Strauss 1975; Yager 1977) have received a great deal of support as effective strategies to manage these issues (Molina 1983–84; Ross and Leichner 1986).

This chapter is organized in a fashion similar to those pertaining to the psychodynamic, biological, and behavioral formulations. It begins with a brief review of the theoretical premises of the biopsychosocial model, describes important underlying formulation principles that affect the model, outlines specific areas of model content, formulates the case of Mr. A, analyzes each step of the formulation, and concludes with a discussion of several implications of the model.

Theoretical Premises of the Biopsychosocial Model

The basic theoretical underpinning of the biopsychosocial model is systems theory as described by von Bertalanffy (1968), Menninger (1963), Engel (1980), Marmor (1983), and others. Engel pointed out that systems theory identifies what to many might seem obvious: nature is organized as a hierarchical continuum from less complex, smaller units such as cells through intermediate units such as individuals and up to more complex, larger units such as societies. Each level in this hierarchy has its own identity and possesses distinct qualities, relationships, and criteria for explanation and study. At the same time, each level is also a component of a higher level. Engel wrote that "every unit is at the very same time both a whole and a part"; an individual "represents at the same time the highest level of the organismic hierarchy and the lowest level of the social hierarchy"; and "every system is influenced by the configuration of the system of which each is a part, that is, by its environment" (p. 537). To understand a system adequately at any level requires both an analysis of its component levels as well as an understanding of its unique characteristics as a system. No level can be understood merely by reducing it to a combination of lower levels. The whole will always be greater then the sum of its parts (Molina 1983–84). Thorough understanding will always require not only a consideration of data from multiple levels but also a process of integrating that data into a unique perspective.

Marmor (1983) described how systems theory applies to human personality and behavior. He uses systems theory to explain how personality develops out of "interactions of the human biological substrate" with influences from the environment, family, school, community, and so on. As a result, a search for the origins of psychopathology must include not only an analysis of what is happening within an individual but also an examination of that person's total system of relationships. Change within any component can produce "ripple effects" throughout the system.

For Marmor (1983), there are profound clinical implications of systems thinking. A systems approach suggests that change at multiple levels within the system might have either positive or negative effects on an individual. Sources of stress do not always come from within or perhaps even close to an individual, and the most effective interventions in any clinical situation might not entail direct involvement of the identified patient. Similarly, to understand the impact of stressful situations on an individual requires an understanding of the context within which the stress occurs. The nature of the system of which the individual is a part, both internal and external, is a major determinant of both the impact of stress and how the individual copes with it.

Nonsystems thinking also yields significant consequences. Marmor (1983) described such an approach as "a tendency to think of causation in linear, unifactorial terms, rather than in terms of the complex pluralistic, multifactorial dynamics that are involved in all human psychopathology" (p. 835). The result of such nonsystems thinking is a form of "reductionism" in which only one aspect of a system is emphasized, be it biological, psychological, sociological, or whatever. Lazare (1989) defined reductionism as "the process by which (and the belief that) various phenomena are explained by mechanisms at a lower level in the scientific hierarchy" (p. 13). To counter a reductionistic approach requires careful consideration of multiple factors at all levels that have contributed to an individual's psychopathology.

Systems theory implies that a broad-based, pluralistic approach is required because of the many factors that contribute to an individual's health or pathology. Yager (1977) arrived at the same conclusion but makes a persuasive argument for "psychiatric eclecticism" to counter the biases inherent in our own "perceptual-cognitive apparatus." This type of eclectic approach entails an analysis of a clinical situation from multiple theoretical perspectives, recognizing the genuine contribution that each point of view can make to understanding a patient but also realizing its limitations as well. The psychiatrist must be open-minded and flexible. The psychiatrist must use the information obtained, including feedback from the patient's perspective, to define and prioritize problems and to suggest a form of therapy that is consistent with the patient's expectations and with what the psychiatrist knows to be most effective and efficient.

Doherty (1989) supports the theoretical value of the biopsychosocial model as a means of understanding the complex interplay of biological, psychological, and social factors in the development of diseases and in their treatment. Doherty also recognizes, however, the practical utility of a "split biopsychosocial model" as a transition between the "radical biomedical" perspective that views diseases and their treatments as reducible to biological processes and the "radical psychosocial" perspective that views diseases and their treatments as strictly psychosocial phenomena. In the split biopsychosocial model, psychosocial factors are recognized as important, but they are not yet integrated with biological factors. Problems are identified as either primarily biological or primarily psychosocial, and their treatments are designed accordingly. The split biopsychosocial model does represent progress toward a synthesis of biological and psychosocial issues but it falls short of a truly integrated biopsychosocial model. Doherty believes that the split biopsychosocial model characterizes the actual practice style of most clinicians who theoretically endorse the biopsychosocial approach.

Molina (1983–84) also noted that the biopsychosocial model has emerged to meet the need for a better understanding of the "human being as a unit, with his biological, psychological and sociological perspectives" (p. 29). He went on to criticize the model, however, for failing to explain the interaction of biological, psychological, and social factors in mental illness. Molina attempts to provide an explanation for this interaction by applying the concepts of "multicausality of illness" and "vulnerability of systems." All illnesses are caused by the interaction of multiple factors, and an understanding of disease must take into consideration the state of vulnerability of the biological, psychological, and social systems prior to the development of the disease process itself. Molina believes that a consideration of these issues will yield a better understanding of the dynamics of the disease process and a better treatment plan.

Abrams (1981, 1983) and Lazare (1989), although also recognizing the strength of the biopsychosocial approach, have noted that it does not identify which of many factors is most important in a given clinical situation, at what level treatment should begin, what treatments should be combined, and when treatments should be changed. Abrams (1983) recommends that the causes of mental illness be viewed in a hierarchy from biological to psychosocial to existential-moral and that treatment should be conducted in a similar "serial" fashion whenever possible.

Lazare (1989) advocates a "multidimensional approach" in which patients are viewed "simultaneously and separately through alternative horizontal and vertical frames of reference" (p. 15). The vertical perspective involves the integration of information from various levels in an individual's system in a manner similar to Engel's (1980) biopsychosocial model. The horizontal perspective entails the integration of explanatory models within a given level on the hierarchy, such as the various schools of thought currently employed to explain psychological phenomena and their treatment. In the multidimensional approach, the psychiatrist uses his or her knowledge, skill, and judgment to employ the most effective and efficient combination of perspectives for patient evaluation and treatment.

Sabelli and Carlson-Sabelli (1989) also are critical of both eclecticism and systems theory as means to integrate biological, social, and psychological factors in psychiatric care. Like Abrams (1981, 1983) and Lazare (1989), they believe eclecticism is insufficient because it does not indicate which factor is most important in a given situation. They fault systems theory for not providing guidelines concerning the sequence in which problems are to be addressed. They find theories advocating a sequential biopsychosocial approach or those implying that treatment can start anywhere in the system to be at variance with the sociobiological perspective, which recognizes that social processes precede an individual's psychological development. For Sabelli and Carlson-Sabelli, process theory that is based on mathematical dynamics yields a comprehensive biosociopsychological method of integrating biological, social, and psychological factors.

Process theory implies that processes are ordered in a hierarchy according to their complexity—biological, social, and psychological. Higher, more complex levels control the function of and thus have supremacy over lower, simpler levels, but simpler processes have priority over more complex, higher levels. For example, biological aspects of mental processes have priority, whereas social and psychological aspects have supremacy. Interventions should be designed in a manner giving priority to biological needs while at the same time recognizing the supremacy of social and psychological factors. Although a person's basic, biological needs should be addressed first, once a measure of stability has occurred, social and psychological needs will quickly become more important treatment issues. The process model is also inherently flexible, however, and recognizes that interventions often must focus on only one particular level at a time. There can be no rigid, fixed formula that can be applied uniformly to every clinical situation.

As noted in Chapter 1, we believe that the theoretical premises of the biopsychosocial hypothesis have evolved to yield the following clinical hypotheses:

1. A patient's problems are best understood in terms of multicausation involving biological, psychological, and sociocultural factors rather than a single etiology.
2. A patient's problems are best understood in terms of the patient's biological, psychological, and sociocultural vulnerabilities.
3. A patient's problems are best understood as manifestations of the patient's attempt to cope with stressors given his or her vulnerabilities and resources.
4. A patient's condition is best treated with a multimodal approach that is flexible and tailored to the patient's needs and expectations rather than with a single treatment modality.

A Comprehensive Biopsychosocial Formulation Model: Underlying Principles and Content

We have previously defined a psychiatric formulation as "a prescribed method for the orderly combination or arrangement of data and treatment recommendations about a psychiatric patient according to some rational principles" (Faulkner et al. 1985, p. 192). This definition underscores the importance of the underlying principles in determining the actual content and process of a formulation model. To understand the approach of a particular model requires an appreciation of its theoretical foundation.

We believe that there are several important underlying principles that combine to determine the content and process of a comprehensive biopsychosocial model (Faulkner et al. 1985). Perhaps most important is the belief that a formulation model must be pluralistic enough to integrate data from all major theoretical perspectives concerning etiology and treatment. In addition, however, it must also enable the clinician to specify the most important factors in any given situation. The model should describe a patient according to a particular format, but it should also be flexible enough to be adapted to a variety of clinical programs, service settings, and patient types. Although based on objective data from psychiatric and medical histories and examinations, the model must also enable the clinician to reach subjective, interpretive conclusions based on the data. Any modern formulation model must be consistent with the multiaxial, cross-sectional, descriptive approach of DSM-III-R (American Psychiatric Association 1987), but it should also incorporate longitudinal, developmental data. It must be a dynamic instrument that evolves as new patient information becomes available. In addition to integrating data from past history and development, the model should also stress an assessment of a patient's current functioning and a delineation of specific problems as well as a treatment plan and a prognosis for the future. A formulation must be detailed enough to provide a thorough understanding of a patient, yet it must also be clear, concise, and relatively easy to produce and read.

Based on a consideration of these formulation principles, we believe that a comprehensive biopsychosocial formulation model should include the following 12 components that are divided somewhat arbitrarily into four categories (Faulkner et al. 1985).

Summary Statement

Case summary. This is a succinct summary of pertinent objective data and subjective impressions derived from a patient evaluation. It includes demographic information, chief complaints, presenting problems, major signs and symptoms, and other important information from the patient's history that will form the basis for the other components in the formulation.

Precipitating stress. This section describes the nature and severity of the specific stressors that might have produced or contributed to the patient's condition. The classic work of Holmes and Rahe (1967) suggests that stressful events can be quantified with respect to the amount of readjustment required for each. Rutter (1981, 1986) clearly articulated the importance of the impact of acute and chronic stress on psychological functioning, but he also emphasized the effects of marked individual differences in constitutional susceptibility, vulnerabilities, and resilience created by early life experiences, protective influences, the social context of the stressful events, and the characteristics of the two-way interaction of the patient with his or her environment. There is no simple relationship between stress and psychiatric illness. Many major threatening events are not followed by disorders, and many disorders are not preceded by any recognized stressful event. Rutter also noted that to understand the effect of stress requires an equal understanding of a person's ability to cope with different events. In turn, coping ability may well be influenced by factors such as a person's age, sex, genetic endowment, temperament, intelligence, psychosocial support network, cognitive appraisal of the stressful event, and the specific process of coping itself.

Patient Characterization

Biological characterization. The major genetic, constitutional, temperamental, and medical factors are listed here. Cantwell and Tarjan (1979) reviewed the relationship of constitutional and organic factors to psychiatric disorders in children. They noted the association in children between psychiatric disorders and brain damage and dysfunction. They also recognized, however, that there does not yet appear to be any specific type of psychiatric disorder that is associated with brain damage in children. Rogoff and Lazare (1989) provided an excellent general review of the contribution of biological factors to psychopathology. They discussed the relationship between medical disease and psychiatric symptoms and the influence of psychological and social factors on biological processes and disease. Meyersburg and Post (1979) suggested ways in which basic psychological constructs such as fixation and regression might be explained by biochemical, physiological, and anatomical processes. They believe there are critical periods for neural development and maturation that underlie human perceptions, cognitions, and affective functions. They hypothesized that "environmental and social experiences may affect both the neural substrates and the subsequent behavior which these neural structures subserve, given the particular state of development of the organism at the time" (p. 150). The contributions of biological factors to a case formulation are described in much greater detail in Chapter 2.

Psychological characterization. This section describes the patient's personality structure and functioning throughout his or her life cycle and includes psychodynamic, behavioral, cognitive, existential, and moral considerations. It includes information about conscious and unconscious conflicts, defense mechanisms, ego functions, maladaptive behavior patterns, cognitive style, object relations, and speculations about possible transference and countertransference reactions. MacKinnon and Yudofsky (1986), Perry et al. (1987), and Alonso (1989) provided good reviews of important psychodynamic issues; Shapiro (1965) described different cognitive styles; and Wolpe and Turkat (1988) and Glynn et al. (1989) outlined important behavioral considerations. Karasu and Skodal (1980) pointed out the limits of DSM-III (American Psychiatric Association 1980) in planning psychotherapy treatment. They noted that a "comprehensive psychodynamic evaluation" requires an assessment of the appropriateness of psychotherapy, the indicated therapeutic approach and its prognosis, the nature of the therapeutic contract, the frequency and duration of treatment, the goals and purpose of psychotherapy, the anticipated nature of the therapeutic relationship and its complications, and the potential transference and countertransference issues. Karasu and Skodal recognized the need for more valid and reliable methods for the evaluation of a patient's conflicts, object relations, defenses, coping mechanisms, and mental structure and proposed that a sixth axis of DSM-III be created to include formal sets of criteria for these psychological issues. The contributions of psychological factors to a case formulation are described more fully in Chapter 2 on the psychodynamic formulation and in Chapter 4 on the behavioral formulation.

Sociocultural characterization. Social and economic class and values, cultural orientation, religious background, social and recreational activities, and interpersonal relationships that contribute to or modify a patient's condition are acknowledged here. Eisenthal (1989) reviewed the influences of sociocultural factors on mental disorders, patienthood, the clinician, and the communication of symptoms. He noted that

> the sociocultural approach will be defined in terms of how the individual functions in his or her social system. Whether or not a person defines him- or herself or is defined by others as "ill" . . . depends not so much on the person's biology, intrapsychic structure, or behavior as on social influences such as the person's status, support systems, sociocultural group, and community. . . . [To be effective] the clinician needs sociocultural data relevant to etiology, entry into the health care system, definition of the problem, orientation and motivation for treatment, treatment expectations, requests for help, maintenance of the disorder, and an individual's potential for engaging in the change process. (p. 70)

Eisenthal (1989) described the effects of social stress and support, social integration and disintegration, and family dynamics on the development of mental dysfunction and disorders. As noted earlier, an understanding of the effects of stress requires information about not only the stressful event but also about the subject involved and the social context within which the stress takes place. The structure and function of the subject's support network can help to mediate the effects of stress. Cohen and Sokolovsky (1979) described a specific method for the analysis of a patient's social network that documents the extent, frequency, duration, intensity, and directional flow of social relationships. This type of analysis has shown that the social networks of psychiatric patients are indeed different from those of normal individuals (Cutler and Tatum 1983).

Loof (1979) used the Southern Appalachian region as a paradigm to illustrate the effects of sociocultural factors on child development, psychopathology, and the healthy aspects of personality functioning. Loof noted that the effects of social class on mental health are "uneven and complex." The clinician must determine whether cultural patterns provide a source of support to growth and development or serve as a negative force to be overcome by the patient.

Familial characterization. Pertinent history of the patient's family of origin and current family structure and function are described in this section. Fleck (1983) outlined nine stages and their associated tasks in the family life cycle: marital, nurturance, toddling, relationship, family unity, adolescence, emancipation, late middle, and aging. He recommended that the axes of DSM-IV be expanded to include personality formulation as well as an assessment of leadership, boundaries, affectivity, communication, and task-goal performance at each stage in the family life cycle. This type of assessment yields a cross-sectional analysis of a family's present functioning as well as a longitudinal view concerning the family's ability to meet the tasks and goals at each stage in its development.

Role performance characterization. This section documents the assets and deficits in a patient's daily living skills and occupational, educational, and recreational roles. When combined with personal, social, and familial information from the other sections, it provides an overview of a patient's psychosocial network (Cutler 1981; Faulkner et al. 1984). This type of information is crucial to the development of an effective treatment plan, especially for patients with chronic mental illnesses. Although many patients will have deficits in multiple roles, most will have a number of strengths as well, and some may possess exceptional talent in a particular area. A treatment plan should include rehabilitation activities that both minimize patient deficits and utilize their assets.

Biopsychosocial Formulation Statement

Integrative statement. A formulation must be more than merely a listing of information about various components (Wallace 1983). It should also identify data that are believed to be most important in a particular clinical situation and proceed to integrate the information together in a meaningful way. There may be many acceptable formats for this integration. Abrams (1983) began with a consideration of biological factors, followed by psychosocial issues, and finally existential-moral considerations; Lazare (1989) attempted to view patient data simultaneously through both vertical and horizontal frames of reference; and Sabelli and Carlson-Sabelli (1989) advocated an approach that considers biological, social, and psychological factors, in that order. We recommend a longitudinal, developmental approach in which the clinician documents his or her understanding of a patient's experience over time. We suggest that pertinent biological characteristics be mentioned first, followed, in order, by important information from familial, sociocultural, psychological, and role performance components. Important life events and precipitating stresses are included at appropriate points of their occurrence. The result is a brief description of how a patient has evolved to his or her present position and level of function.

Diagnosis, Problem List, Treatment Plan, and Prognosis

DSM-III-R diagnosis and differential diagnosis. Information from previous sections is summarized here in a formal, multiaxial DSM-III-R diagnosis. Mezzich et al. (1982) suggested a useful format for listing principal, provisional, and alternative diagnoses to be considered on Axes I, II, and III; ranking and rating the severity of psychosocial stressors on Axis IV; and rating the highest level of adaptive functioning during the past year on Axis V.

Problem list. As a result of the comprehensive analysis of information in the previous sections, specific medical, intrapsychic, and psychosocial network problems are identified. As much as possible, the therapist and patient should reach a consensus about what specific problems exist, since they will need to work together to attempt to manage them (Lazare 1989; Yager 1977). Anthony (1979) recognized the limits of the traditional psychiatric diagnosis in predicting the results of treatment and rehabilitation. He recommended a rehabilitation diagnosis that includes information about a patient's current abilities and what will be expected of the patient by the community in which he or she will need to function. These data enable the clinician to develop a problem list and a treatment plan that increase a patient's strengths and also identify the setting most suitable for the patient. Anthony's three-stage "rehabilitation approach to diagnosis" includes the exploration, understanding, and assessment of the patient and his or her problems and goals in living, learning, and working environments. Whatever problem list is developed should be considered to be a dynamic instrument to be modified as changes occur in the patient's condition or circumstances.

Treatment plan. Once problems have been identified, a specific treatment plan is developed to address them. Again, as much as possible, there should be consensus between therapist and patient. Specific medications, psychotherapy, and practical psychosocial network interventions are listed in this section (Cutler et al. 1983). The literature suggests a considerable divergence of opinion concerning the order in which treatment methods should be applied. Engel's (1980) approach is biopsychosocial; Abrams' (1983) is "biopsychosocioexistential-moral"; Yager's (1977) and Lazare's (1989) are eclectic, pluralistic, and multidimensional; and Sabelli and Carlson-Sabelli's (1989) is biosociopsychological. Pribram (1981) believes that treatment can begin at any point in a system since all parts are interconnected. Each of these authors is a strong advocate for his or her perspective, but a close reading of their work reveals that they also emphasize the importance of flexibility in the approach to any specific clinical situation. In general, we suggest that clinicians proceed from biological to psychosocial issues, but practical realities will often determine the order of treatment. Like the problem list, the treatment plan is also a dynamic instrument that should be modified to take into consideration any changes that occur in the patient's situation.

Prognosis. This section contains a statement of the patient's prognosis and expected treatment response. This will usually be determined by a combination of factors, including the patient's diagnosis, past history, previous level of functioning, current life situation, natural history of his or her disorder, his or her desire for change, and the competence of his or her clinician. The prognosis for many disorders is still unknown, but DSM-III-R does contain information on conditions such as schizophrenia and affective disorders.

Each of the sections above lists the type of specific information we believe the formulation components should include along with references that suggest ways of organizing and presenting the data. We do not mean to imply that these are the only acceptable formats. Each component has been the subject of extensive investigation from many different perspectives. To us, the manner in which data are organized in each component is less important than ensuring that all components are included and that consideration is given to how the components are integrated to produce a comprehensive formulation.

Formulation of the Case of Mr. A

Summary Statement

Case summary. Mr. A is a 42-year-old married businessman with two children, a 12-year-old girl and a 10-year-old boy, who presents with complaints of loss of interest in his job, hobbies, and family over a 6-week period after he was passed over for a job promotion. He also has problems of profound sadness, decreased appetite and weight loss, insomnia, fatigue, and recurrent thoughts of death. Mr. A has no history of manic or psychotic symptoms, suicidal or homicidal ideations, substance abuse, medical problems, or psychiatric treatment. He is a serious, conservative, perfectionist, controlling, and hard-working person who has trouble expressing affection. Mr. A has had marital problems for several years. His wife had withdrawn from him emotionally and sexually until his recent problems, which have prompted her attention and concern. Mr. A comes from an impoverished background. His father deserted the family when he was 12, and he had to help rear his younger siblings and work to support the family and put himself through school. There is a family history of alcoholism, suicide, and sociopathy.

Precipitating stress. The major stressors for Mr. A appear to be his recent failure to be promoted, chronic marital problems, and the emotional and sexual withdrawal (i.e., abandonment) by his wife. The fact that his children are nearing the age of independence and are near the age when he experienced a significant trauma in his own life (i.e., the desertion of his father) may also represent significant stressors.

Patient Characterization

Biological characterization. Mr. A's family history of alcoholism, suicide, and sociopathy makes it likely that he has a genetic predisposition for affective illness. His affective, cognitive, behavioral, and vegetative symptoms are indicative of an endogenous type of depression.

Psychological characterization. Mr. A appears to have major conflicts over dependency and autonomy. Because of his earlier experience with significant loss, the withdrawal of attention and affection by Mr. A's wife, the growing independence of his children, and being passed over for promotion represent significant precipitating events. Mr. A has considerable difficulty expressing emotions and affection. He is controlling and perfectionist. He views himself as inadequate, defective, and unlovable. His cognitive style is obsessive-compulsive. His primary defenses are repression, regression, introjection, isolation of affect, and intellectualization. Psychotherapy for Mr. A would be complicated by his cognitive style and his conflicts over dependency and autonomy.

Sociocultural characterization. Mr. A's sociocultural background has helped to instill in him a basic belief in the value of hard work, stoicism, and self-reliance with little dependence on extrafamilial sources of support. From a young age, he has been reinforced to sacrifice himself and to maintain the role of provider and nurturer to others who have depended on him for support.

Familial characterization. Mr. A is distant from his family of origin, and his current life centers around his immediate family. His role has been as a provider to a wife and children who have been dependent on him. Mr. A and his wife have not been able to form a satisfactory marital coalition, they do few things together, and their sexual relationship has deteriorated. His wife has withdrawn in the last few years, and his children now are nearing independence.

Role performance characterization. Mr. A has been able to adapt fairly well educationally and occupationally. He has been able to work productively as a businessman. However, he has limited social relationships, no close friends, and few independent recreational activities.

Biopsychosocial Formulation Statement

Integrative statement. Mr. A's probable biological predisposition to affective instability, coupled with the abandonment by his father, familial modeling, sociocultural reinforcement, and negative cognitive schemata resulted in the development of an inadequate, defective, and unlovable self-concept and a rigid, obsessive-compulsive personality. His role evolved into one of stoic, hard-working self-sacrifice in the service of others who are dependent on him and a denial of his own dependency and autonomy needs. While adaptive educationally and occupationally, his personality structure and ego defenses resulted in an isolated life-style and the inability to acknowledge his own feelings or to relate to others with warmth and affection. The symbolic abandonment by his wife and children and his failure at work reawakened old dependency and autonomy conflicts, threatened his adaptive role in life, overwhelmed his rigid defenses, and resulted in anxiety, regression, and depression.

DSM-III-R Diagnosis and Differential Diagnosis

Axis I Major depression, single episode (296.22)
Axis II Obsessive-compulsive personality disorder (301.40)
Axis III No diagnosis
Axis IV Severity of Psychosocial Stressors: 3, with moderate stress due to marital discord
Axis V Current Global Assessment of Functioning (GAF) score: 52; highest GAF score past year: 67

Problem List

1. Depression
   Insomnia
   Decreased appetite and weight loss
   Decreased interest

Fatigue
Thoughts of death
2. Marital discord
Lack of emotional closeness
Sexual difficulties
3. Obsessive-compulsive personality disorder
Isolation of affect
Difficulty expressing affection
4. Limited social relationships with no friends
5. Limited recreational activities

Treatment Plan

1. Antidepressant medication
2. Supportive psychotherapy evolving to insight-oriented therapy as depressive symptoms abate (group therapy)
3. Marital therapy (sexual therapy)
4. Social and recreational activities

Prognosis

Since this is a single, discrete episode of depression in a person with good premorbid functioning, the prognosis for a return to a baseline level is good. It is likely that Mr. A's depressive symptom will respond to medication. His obsessive-compulsive personality disorder and unmet dependency needs are long-standing problems with a more guarded prognosis that depends on his ability to engage in effective psychotherapy and to expand and modify his range of contacts and activities. The prognosis for his marriage is also guarded and depends on the willingness of his wife and himself to examine their relationship, explore new avenues of interaction, and modify their roles. Marital therapy will likely be required to accomplish these goals.

Step-by-Step Analysis of the Case Formulation

This part of the chapter is included to illustrate how the formulation of the case of Mr. A was developed. Each section of the formulation will be considered in turn.

Summary Statement

This section includes a brief case summary and a listing of those life events that might represent precipitating stressors. The case summary for Mr. A merely restates those aspects of his history that will need to be considered and explained in later sections of the formulation.

The precipitating stressors that have been suggested for Mr. A are those events we believe might have had a major impact on his psychological equilibrium given his personality structure, vulnerabilities, and resources. It is not always clear just exactly what represents a significant precipitating event for a given patient. Incidents that appear to be minor to one person can have great symbolic meaning for another, and other events that might be expected to be very disturbing are sometimes managed with remarkable ease. A clinician is best advised to take his or her lead from the patient as to whether or not a stress has occurred and then strive to understand the meaning of the stressor to the patient and his or her response to it. In the case of Mr. A, we have hypothesized that job and marital difficulties represent stressors and suggest that developmental issues with his children might also be significant precipitating events in his life. There is clear evidence to support the traumatic impact of occupational and marital difficulties on psychological stability (Holmes and Rahe 1967; Rutter 1981). Although perhaps supported by less objective evidence, many clinicians have also noted that children can serve as potent reminders to parents of important developmental issues in their own lives (Lidz 1976).

Patient Characterization

This section generally follows the approach endorsed by Lazare (1989), Yager (1977), and others and considers the data available on Mr. A from multiple perspectives. This helps to prevent an overemphasis on any one particular aspect of Mr. A, and it also makes it more likely that a variety of treatment interventions will be revealed in the process. Since the case of Mr. A has been presented very schematically as an example, limited data are available. This makes our analysis somewhat superficial and very tentative. Based on what we do know, however, we are able to outline important considerations in each subsection for Mr. A.

In the biological subsection, we note Mr. A's genetic loading for affective illness (Nurnberger and Gershon 1984) and his symptoms, which suggest an endogenous type of depression (Klein et al. 1980). This information will be crucial to whatever decisions are made about psychotropic medication for Mr. A.

Because of the multitude of different theoretical perspectives pertaining to it, the psychological subsection can be the most difficult and controversial to describe. Many clinicians endorse one particular model as a framework to interpret psychological data, whereas others are more pluralistic in their approach (Lazare 1989; Perry et al. 1987). We support the latter point of view. Using the data available on Mr. A, in this subsection we describe what appears to be his major conflicts, defense mechanisms, cognitive style and schemata, and possible transference and countertransference issues. Much more information would be needed to understand fully Mr. A's dynamic, behavioral, object relations, and existential-moral issues.

From the limited sociocultural data available on Mr. A, we are able to infer a few things about how he seems to function in his social system and postulate why that might be so. The richness of a person's social network and the availability of emotional support do appear to be factors that help determine his or her response to stress (Cohen and Sokolovsky 1979; Eisenthal 1989). It does seem that Mr. A has few external sources of support to help him deal with his current difficulties. We have no information, however, about his religious beliefs or the nature of his interaction with friends or extended family.

In the familial characterization, we attempt to describe how Mr. A and his wife function as a couple and as parents. Although it appears that he has been able to provide adequately for his family, there is some evidence to suggest that Mr. A has not been able to meet the emotional needs of his wife. It appears that the two of them have not been able to function together as a unit to support one another or to evolve their family through a constructive, developmental life cycle that will help them meet the challenges that lie ahead (Fleck 1983).

The role performance subsection provides us with an opportunity to note how Mr. A appears to perform in a variety of different roles with different responsibilities and pressures. This type of analysis is crucial to a thorough understanding of Mr. A's strengths that can be used to his benefit and deficits that need to be addressed in his treatment plan (Faulkner et al. 1984).

Biopsychosocial Formulation Statement

This section integrates data from the preceding two sections in a manner that will provide an overall picture of how Mr. A has evolved to his current position and level of function. We begin by acknowledging Mr. A's biological factors. We then note in order his pertinent familial, sociocultural, and psychological considerations. We describe the impact of these issues on

Mr. A's role performance and conclude by illustrating the effect of current stressors on his psychological equilibrium.

As we stated earlier, there may be many acceptable ways to integrate clinical data together (Abrams 1983; Lazare 1989; Sabelli and Carlson-Sabelli 1989). There is not necessarily one correct method. The approach that we have described here, however, makes sense to us because it seems to follow a path that parallels human development. A child begins with a biological substrate, evolves a personality under the influence of family and society, and proceeds to fulfill a variety of roles. The impact of stressful events can be appreciated only in the context of the patient's biological, familial, social, psychological, and role performance resources and vulnerabilities.

Diagnosis, Problem List, Treatment Plan, and Prognosis

The diagnostic subsection is relatively straightforward and conforms to the five axes of DSM-III-R. The problem list uses information derived from the summary statement, patient characterization, and biopsychosocial formulation statement as well as the diagnostic subsection to clarify specific issues that need to be addressed in Mr. A's treatment plan. We note that Mr. A's problem list contains items that were brought to light in the process of analyzing his situation from multiple perspectives. It identifies biological, familial, psychological, social, and role performance difficulties that need to be considered. Mr. A's treatment plan provides an overview of a possible approach to the management of his problems in each of these areas. We have only sketched an outline of the elements that might be included in Mr. A's treatment. Each component could obviously be described in great detail. This might become necessary if Mr. A fails to respond to rather straightforward interventions or if untoward complications arise. The prognostic subsection presents our prediction about how Mr. A will likely respond to his treatment plan. It is based on our knowledge of Mr. A's prior level of functioning, a consideration of the natural history of his disorders, the demonstrated effectiveness of the treatments we have suggested, and our sense about his willingness to cooperate with our therapy. We note that the prognosis for the resolution of Mr. A's acute difficulties is more favorable than for the modification of his more lifelong patterns of behavior.

Discussion

There are several important clinical and educational implications of a comprehensive biopsychosocial formulation model like the one described here

(Faulkner et al. 1985). First, it accommodates different theoretical approaches to patients and has wide applicability to different service settings. The same formulation can follow patients as they move throughout a clinical service network from inpatient wards to outpatient clinics.

Second, the model's components and organization help ensure that broad-based, thorough clinical evaluations are done on every patient and that one's own cognitive bias does not interfere with assessments. By linking together the patient characterization and formulation statement with the diagnosis, problem list, and treatment plan, the model provides both in-depth knowledge as well as practical, clinically relevant information.

Third, the model provides a structure to help guide trainees as they evaluate patients and an organizational framework within which to integrate and balance new knowledge they acquire about the various model components. It encourages both trainees and faculty to take a more pluralistic, comprehensive approach to patients. It also enables faculty to emphasize their own theoretical perspective and to demonstrate to trainees how their orientation can contribute to the understanding of specific patients.

The process of constructing a formulation is always a difficult task because patients themselves are so complicated. The content and process of a comprehensive biopsychosocial formulation model, however, can be used as an effective tool to increase understanding about patients and produce a rational approach to treatment.

References

Abrams EM: Beyond eclecticism. Am J Psychiatry 140:740–745, 1983

Abrams GM: Psychiatric serialism. Compr Psychiatry 22:372–378, 1981

Alonso A: The psychodynamic approach, in Outpatient Psychiatry Diagnosis and Treatment, 2nd Edition. Edited by Lazare A. Baltimore, MD, Williams & Wilkins, 1989, pp 37–58

American Psychiatric Association: Diagnostic and Statistical Manual of Mental Disorders, 3rd Edition. Washington, DC, American Psychiatric Association, 1980

American Psychiatric Association: Diagnostic and Statistical Manual of Mental Disorders, 3rd Edition, Revised. Washington, DC, American Psychiatric Association, 1987

American Psychiatric Association: Diagnostic and Statistical Manual of Mental Disorders, 4th Edition, First Draft. Washington, DC, American Psychiatric Association, 1991

Anthony WA: The rehabilitation approach to diagnosis. New Dir Ment Health Serv 2:25–36, 1979

Cantwell DP, Tarjan G: Constitutional-organic factors in etiology, in Basic Handbook of Child Psychiatry. Edited by Noshpitz JD. New York, Basic Books, 1979, pp 28–62

Cleghorn JM: Formulation: a pedagogic antidote to DSM-III. Compr Psychiatry 26:504–512, 1985

Cohen CI, Sokolovsky J: Clinical use of network analysis for psychiatric and aged populations. Community Ment Health J 15:203–213, 1979

Cummings JL: Neuropsychiatry: the paradigm shift. The Psychiatric Times, January 1990, pp 41–43

Cutler DL: The chronically mentally ill, in Community Mental Health: A Sourcebook for Professionals and Advisory Board Members. Edited by Silverman WH. New York, Praeger, 1981, pp 344–358

Cutler DL, Tatum E: Networks and the chronic patient. New Dir Ment Health Serv 19:13–22, 1983

Cutler DL, Terwilliger WB, Faulkner LR: Integrating an aftercare plan for the chronic patient. New Dir Ment Health Serv 19:95–104, 1983

Doherty WJ: Challenges to integration: research and clinical issues, in Family Systems in Medicine. Edited by Ramsey LN. New York, Guilford, 1989, pp 571–582

Eisenthal S: The sociocultural approach, in Outpatient Psychiatry Diagnosis and Treatment, 2nd Edition. Edited by Lazare A. Baltimore, MD, Williams & Wilkins, 1989, pp 69–102

Engel GL: The clinical application of the biopsychosocial model. Am J Psychiatry 137:535–544, 1980

Faulkner LR, Terwilliger WB, Cutler DL: Productive activities for the chronic patient. Community Ment Health J 20:109–122, 1984

Faulkner LR, Kinzie JD, Angell R, et al: A comprehensive psychiatric formulation model. Journal of Psychiatric Education 9:189–203, 1985

Fink PJ: Response to the presidential address: is "biopsychosocial" the psychiatric shibboleth? Am J Psychiatry 145:1061–1067, 1988

Fleck S: A holistic approach to family typology and the axes of DSM-III. Arch Gen Psychiatry 40:901–906, 1983

Glynn SM, Mueser KT, Liberman RP: The behavioral approach, in Outpatient Psychiatry Diagnosis and Treatment, 2nd Edition. Edited by Lazare A. Baltimore, MD, Williams & Wilkins, 1989, pp 59–68

Goldsmith SR, Mandell AJ: The dynamic formulation: a critique of a psychiatric ritual. Am J Psychiatry 125:152–157, 1969

Holmes T, Rahe RH: The social readjustment rating scale. J Psychosom Res 11:213–218, 1967

Karasu TB, Skodal AE: VIth axis for DSM-III: psychodynamic evaluation. Am J Psychiatry 137:607–610, 1980

Klein DF, Gittelman R, Quitkin F, et al (eds): Diagnosis of affective disorders: clinical considerations, in Diagnosis and Drug Treatment of Psychiatric Disorders: Adults and Children, 2nd Edition. Baltimore, MD, Williams & Wilkins, 1980, pp 223–250

Kline S, Cameron PM: I: Formulation. Canadian Psychiatric Association Journal 23:39–42, 1978

Lazare A: A multidimensional approach to psychopathology, in Outpatient Psychiatry Diagnosis and Treatment, 2nd Edition. Edited by Lazare A. Baltimore, MD, Williams & Wilkins, 1989, pp 7–16

Lidz T: The Person: His and Her Development Throughout the Life Cycle. New York, Basic Books, 1976

Loof D: Sociocultural factors in etiology, in Basic Handbook of Child Psychiatry. Edited by Noshpitz JD. New York, Basic Books, 1979, pp 87–99

MacKinnon RA, Yudofsky SC: DSM-III diagnosis and the psycho-dynamic case formulation, in The Psychiatric Evaluation in Clinical Practice. Edited by MacKinnon RA, Yudofsky SC. Philadelphia, PA, JB Lippincott, 1986, pp 213–250

Marmor J: Systems thinking in psychiatry: some theoretical and clinical implications. Am J Psychiatry 140:833–838, 1983

Menninger K: The Vital Balance. New York, Viking Press, 1963

Meyersburg HA, Post RM: An holistic developmental view of neural and psychological processes: a neurobiological-psychoanalytic integration. Br J Psychiatry 135:139–155, 1979

Mezzich JE, Coffman GA, Goodpastor SM: A format for DSM-III diagnostic formulation: experience with 1,111 consecutive patients. Am J Psychiatry 139:591–596, 1982

Molina JA: Understanding the biopsychosocial model. Int J Psychiatry Med 13:29–36, 1983–84

Nurnberger JI Jr, Gershon ES: Genetics of affective disorders, in Neurobiology of Mood Disorders. Edited by Post R, Ballenger J. Baltimore, MD, Williams & Wilkins, 1984, pp 76–101

Perry S, Cooper AM, Michels R: The psychodynamic formulation: its purpose, structure and clinical application. Am J Psychiatry 144:543–550, 1987

Pribram KH: The neurobiologic paradigm, in Models for Clinical Psychopathology. Edited by Eisdorfer C, Cohen D, Kleinman A, et al. New York, Spectrum Publications, 1981, pp 121–132

Rogoff M, Lazare A: The biologic approach, in Outpatient Psychiatry Diagnosis and Treatment, 2nd Edition. Edited by Lazare A. Baltimore, MD, Williams & Wilkins, 1989, pp 17–36

Ross CA, Leichner P: Canadian and British opinion on formulation. Annals of the Royal College of Physicians and Surgeons of Canada 19:49–52, 1986

Rutter M: Stress, coping, and development: some issues and some questions. J Child Psychol Psychiatry 22:323–356, 1981

Rutter M: Meyerian psychobiology, personality development, and the role of life experiences. Am J Psychiatry 143:1077–1086, 1986

Sabelli HC, Carlson-Sabelli L: Biological priority and psychological supremacy: a new integrative paradigm derived from process theory. Am J Psychiatry 146:1541–1551, 1989

Shapiro D: Neurotic Styles. New York, Basic Books, 1965

Sharfstein SS, Beigel A (eds): The New Economics and Psychiatric Care. Washington, DC, American Psychiatric Press, 1985

Sperry L: Designing effective psychiatric interventions. Journal of Psychiatric Education 12:125–128, 1988

Strauss JS: A comprehensive approach to psychiatric diagnosis. Am J Psychiatry 132:1193–1197, 1975

von Bertalanffy L: General Systems Theory. New York, Braziller, 1968

Wallace ER: Dynamic Psychiatry in Theory and Practice. Philadelphia, PA, Lea & Febiger, 1983

Wolpe J, Turkat ID: Behavioral formulation of clinical cases, in Behavioral Case Formulations. Edited by Turket ID. New York, Harper & Row, 1988, pp 5–36

Yager J: Psychiatric eclecticism: a cognitive view. Am J Psychiatry 134:736–741, 1977

CHAPTER 6

Converging Perspectives on Case Formulations

THE DEVELOPMENT OF FORMULATIONS has a long history in psychiatric education and clinical practice (Cleghorn 1985; Faulkner et al. 1985). In the past, there has been considerable disagreement, however, about what should be included in a formulation and how it should be constructed (Goldsmith and Mandell 1969; Ross and Leichner 1986). As noted in Chapter 1, it appears that there has been a recent convergence of opinion about formulations and perhaps a movement toward a formal integration of perspectives (Abrams 1983; Engle 1980; Lazare 1989; Sabelli and Carlson-Sabelli 1989; Yager 1977). This evolution is in line with the paradigm shift that has taken place in psychiatry over the last three decades as the field has moved from an emphasis on psychoanalysis to a more balanced, biopsychosocial point of view (Abrams 1981; Fink 1988).

In this chapter, we focus on several aspects of the converging perspectives on case formulation. We begin with an analysis of some of the theoretical issues pertaining to the synthesis and integration of clinical data from different perspectives; describe the convergence of different formulation models from the standpoints of their structure, process, and content; and conclude with a brief discussion of some important implications of the convergence of opinion about psychiatric formulations.

The Integration of Clinical Data: Vertical and Horizontal Perspectives

Lazare (1989) described the analysis of patient data using both vertical and horizontal integration. He noted that vertical reasoning "refers to thinking about the objects and processes under study in descending or ascending order according to the size and complexity of the units" (p. 13). This type of approach readily leads to "reductionism," which Lazare defined as "the process by which (and the belief that) various phenomena are explained by mechanisms at a lower level in the scientific hierarchy" (p. 13). In this manner, social processes are explained by psychological mechanisms, and psychological phenomena are explained by biological processes.

Significant problems arise, however, in the application of vertical, reductionistic reasoning to clinical psychiatry. Understanding most psychiatric conditions requires the simultaneous consideration of biological, psychological, and social factors. In addition, many conditions can be understood only by an analysis of higher, rather than lower, levels on a vertical hierarchy. Finally, no level can be understood merely by reducing it to a combination of lower levels. Each level has unique characteristics that emerge as it is formed and evolves. Dissatisfaction with reductionism and the need to explain the emergence of new characteristics unique to each level are factors that have prompted many investigators to focus on concepts of biological and psychosocial integration (Meyersburg and Post 1979), general systems theory (Engel 1980; von Bertalanffy 1968), and, more recently, process theory (Sabelli and Carlson-Sabelli 1989) as means to synthesize clinical data from different vertical levels. Doherty (1989) endorsed general systems theory and the biopsychosocial model for the integration of data on a vertical hierarchy, but he also realized that such a perspective is unlikely to become a reality until practitioners have embraced radical paradigm shifts away from their idiosyncratic points of view. Doherty proposed a "split biopsychosocial model" as a transition between the "radical biomedical" and "radical psychosocial" models and the true biopsychosocial model. The split biopsychosocial model recognizes the value of both biological and psychological issues but does not yet integrate them.

For Lazare (1989), horizontal integration is the process of combining different explanatory models for a particular level on a vertical hierarchy. The proliferation of models is most obvious on the psychological level, where psychodynamic, behavioral, existential, and other models compete, but multiple models have been invoked to explain biological (Rogoff and Lazare 1989) and sociocultural (Eisenthal 1989) phenomena as well. There are also various submodels within each level. For example, the behavioral model includes conditioning as well as cognitive paradigms (Glynn et al. 1989), whereas the psychodynamic model includes ego psychological, self psychological, and object relations perspectives (Perry et al. 1987).

Walsh and Peterson (1985) discussed the attempt at horizontal synthesis of different theoretical perspectives by "single-school expansion" and "cross-school integration." Single-school expansionists broaden the concepts of their particular model to incorporate other perspectives while maintaining their model's traditional approach. Cross-school integrationists combine the strengths of different models into what they believe is a new, better model. Although there have been numerous attempts to integrate models (Beitman et al. 1989; Blanck and Blanck 1979; Marmor and Woods 1980), Walsh and Peterson believe that true synthesis, at least on the psychological level of a vertical hierarchy, is unlikely at this time due to radical methodological differences that exist between current models. They advocated an approach of "pluralism" in which the various theories are kept relatively "pure" and "premature eclecticism" is avoided. Such a pluralistic approach would retain all the major content areas of the various models on a particular horizontal level; encourage cross-fertilization of ideas; stimulate cooperative, cross-school competition; and recognize the strengths and limitations of each model. This position with respect to horizontal integration is similar to Doherty's (1989) on vertical integration: different models are retained as valuable contributors of knowledge but not yet synthesized into an acceptable meta-theory.

Walsh and Peterson's (1985) advocacy for a pluralistic position received considerable support from Lazare (1989), who found fault with systems theory's attempt at vertical integration as well as various horizontal integration efforts. Lazare advocated a "multidimensional approach" in which a clinician attempts to understand a patient's problems "simultaneously and separately through alternative horizontal and vertical frames of reference" (p. 15). Lazare's ideas are very similar to Yager's (1977) "psychiatric eclecticism," in which each clinical situation is approached from multiple theoretical perspectives partly to compensate for the clinician's own perceptual cognitive bias. Abrams's (1981, 1983) "psychiatric serialism" and Sabelli and Carlson-Sabelli's (1989) "biosociopsychological method" are additional examples of comprehensive perspectives that emphasize the consideration of data from multiple vertical levels and horizontal schools of thought.

Although this review of some of the theoretical issues pertaining to the synthesis of clinical data fails to identify a uniformly accepted method for integrating vertical or horizontal information into a comprehensive formulation, it does begin to reveal a convergence of current opinion about aspects of formulation structure, process, and content. The term *convergence* is used here to refer to the emerging similarities among distinct formulation models rather than to an actual integration or synthesis of those models (Beitman et al. 1989). This is akin to the joining together of tributaries to make a larger river. As the streams converge at their point of confluence, their contents flow together but are still separate parts of what might be called a new "eclectic" river. This separation of water in the river will continue until the mixing process can integrate the parts into a uniform body of water. We believe that American psychiatry is today at the point of convergence and eclecticism but some distance yet from total integration.

Formulation Structure and Process

In this book, we focus on four major psychiatric formulation orientations: psychodynamic, biological, behavioral, and biopsychosocial. As shown in Table 1–1 in Chapter 1, these four formulation models can be arranged to reveal similar structure and process. Each model contains sections that summarize the available data and events, try to synthesize the data in a meaningful way, and present treatment options. Each model addresses descriptive, explanatory, and treatment-prognostic issues. Each model asks and attempts to answer, "What happened?," "Why did it happen?," and "What can be done about it and how?" Each formulation moves in sequence from a statement of the pertinent data, to an attempt to explain the meaning of the data, and finally to recommendations about specific treatment based on that understanding.

This convergence of opinion about formulation structure and process is also supported in recent writings about the different models. Lazare (1989) stated that "the clinician using the biologic approach is concerned with etiology, pathogenesis, signs and symptoms, differential diagnosis, treatment, and prognosis" (p. 9). Perry et al. (1987) recommended that a psychodynamic formulation move from a presentation of "a summary of the case" and "a description of nondynamic factors that may have contributed," to "a psychodynamic explanation of the central conflicts," and conclude with "a prediction of how these conflicts are likely to affect treatment" (p. 544). MacKinnon and Yudofsky's (1986) outline of their psychodynamic case formulation is somewhat more extensive than that of Perry et al. (1987) and evolves from a description of the patient, present illness, psychopathology, and developmental data; to a consideration of key psychodynamics and a diagnostic classification that is compatible with DSM-III-R (American Psychiatric Association 1987); and finally to a discussion of transference and countertransference issues, treatment planning, and prognosis. Wolpe and Turkat's (1988) behavioral formulation begins with the collection of data from the interview, "so that a formulation of the presenting problems can be developed." This is followed by "clinical experimentation which aims to validate the formulation" and the development from the formulation of a "modification methodology" that is "implemented and monitored for its efficacy" (p. 7). Lazare (1989) described the behavioral approach as beginning with a determination of "the behaviors to be modified," "the conditions under which the behaviors occur," and "the factors responsible for the persistence of the behaviors." Subsequently, a "set of treatment conditions" is selected and a "schedule of retraining" is arranged (p. 11). Kline and Cameron's (1978) suggested process for a biopsychosocial formulation commences with "longitudinal data collection" and "descriptive cross-sectional evaluation," then moves to "an integrative evaluation including differential diagnosis," and concludes with "a tentative prognosis" (p. 39). Faulkner et al.'s (1985) comprehensive, biopsychosocial formulation model begins with a documentation of case data, stressors, and a multifactorial characterization of the patient; proceeds to an integrative statement that ties the information about the patient together; and concludes with a formal diagnosis, problem list, treatment plan, and statement of prognosis.

In this volume, in Chapter 2, on the psychodynamic formulation, a case formulation is defined as

> a summary of a series of clinical observations that serves as a preparation for therapeutic intervention. It is the process of linking a group of data and information to define a coherent pattern. It helps establish diagnosis, provides for explanation, prepares the clinician for therapeutic work, and provides for therapeutic prediction. (p. 22)

In Chapter 3, on the biological formulation, formulation is defined as

> a succinct statement that encapsulates the etiology, evolution, diagnosis, treatment options, and future prognosis for the patient's problem. (p. 49)

In Chapter 4, on the behavioral formulation, a formulation is described in the conditioning paradigm as

> a hypothesis that 1) relates all of the presenting complaints to one another, 2) explains why these difficulties have developed, and 3) provides predictions of the patient's behavior given any stimulus conditions. (p. 79)

It is also suggested that

> in the cognitive-behavioral paradigm, a formulation is a hypothesis about underlying deficits producing the patient's problems. The formulation serves as the clinician's compass, guiding treatment planning and intervention. . . . [It] can guide the choice of treatment, modality, intervention

> strategy, and point of intervention as well as predict and manage noncompliance. (p. 82–83)

In Chapter 5, on the biopsychosocial formulation, a psychiatric formulation includes the "orderly combination or arrangement of data and treatment recommendations about a psychiatric patient" beginning with a "summary statement" and proceeding through sections that address "patient characterization," a "biopsychosocial formulation statement," and, finally, "diagnosis, problem list, treatment plan, and prognosis."

Formulation Content

An analysis of the content in each section of the four formulation models reveals differences in emphasis but also some striking similarities. In the formulation of the case of Mr. A, each model recognizes the importance of data in the biological, psychological, and social spheres; arrives at a diagnosis that is compatible with DSM-III-R; advocates treatment with medications as well as some type of psychotherapy; and attempts to predict the possible outcome of treatment.

A review of the recent literature on the four formulation models also reveals considerable convergence of opinion about formulation content. In discussing the biological approach to patients, Rogoff and Lazare (1989) noted that

> psychiatrists who have expertise in the biological approach . . . determine what is wrong with the patient by simultaneously considering biologic with other social and psychologic approaches. . . . [and] limiting psychiatric procedures to symptom and syndromal diagnoses and their biologic treatments is ineffective clinical practice. Such a practice will fail in developing and maintaining a therapeutic relationship and in addressing many of the patient's psychologic problems. (p. 33)

In their article on psychodynamic formulation, Perry et al. (1987) reserved an entire section of their model for a consideration of "nondynamic factors." They stated that "a psychodynamic formulation does not ignore the effect of nondynamic factors on the patient's mood, thoughts, and behavior. The dynamic formulation is consistent with the biopsychosocial model, is relevant to all forms of psychiatric treatment" (p. 546). Also writing about the psychodynamic approach to patients, Alonso (1989) indicated that "the clinician must come to terms with biologic, sociocultural, behavioral, and psychodynamic approaches to interpreting clinical data and planning treatment" (p. 50). Glynn et al. (1989) pointed out in their behavioral approach to patients that

> most abnormal behavior is assumed to be acquired and maintained through . . . biopsychosocial mechanisms. . . . It is unlikely that any one set of general principles will very satisfactorily explain the onset, duration, and amelioration or remission of psychiatric problems. . . . Many different biologic and environmental factors are responsible and many different biologic and environmental interventions will be necessary. (pp. 60, 67)

Molina (1983–84) suggested that

> when studying disease under the biopsychosocial model we have to take into consideration the state of vulnerability of the biological, psychological and social systems previous to the development of the disease process. This will enable us to understand its dynamics and develop a better treatment plan. (p. 32)

In this volume, in Chapter 2, on the psychodynamic formulation, we wrote,

> All psychiatrists, regardless of theoretical orientation, should be able to gather anamnestic, descriptive data about the patient's chief complaint; present illness; development; family, social, educational, and work history; medical status; and mental status. . . . It should be clear from the onset that it is not the intention to divide interviewing arbitrarily or artificially into biological, psychodynamic, behavioral (cognitive), and biopsychosocial components, because all must be considered. (p. 22)

In Chapter 3, on the biological formulation, we warned against the "rigid adherence to only a single approach when both medication and psychotherapy would have been indicated" (p. 58). It is suggested that a formulation should capture "the essence of each person's predicament" and "transcend the descriptive parsimony of DSM-III-R by portraying a complete biopsychosocial perspective" (p. 49).

In Chapter 4, on the behavioral formulation, it is noted that a patient's problems

> might include depression, insomnia, panic attacks, eating problems, procrastination, drug and alcohol abuse, phobias, obsessive thoughts, rituals, memory problems, marital conflicts, social isolation, unemployment, housing problems, financial difficulties, headaches, and other medical problems. Even though the patient may resist providing a comprehensive

> listing of concerns, the clinician cannot hope to formulate the case accurately or to intervene successfully without an inclusive list. (p. 83)

In Chapter 5, on the biopsychosocial formulation, we stated that

> the virtual explosion of well-documented data pertaining to the importance of biological, psychological, behavioral, and sociocultural factors in psychiatric diseases and their treatments has made a rigid, reductionistic adherence to one theoretical point of view untenable. (p. 97)

Discussion

There are several important implications of the current state of convergence of opinion about case formulations that warrant discussion. First, similarities in formulation structure, process, and content provide a common framework within which to discuss legitimate differences between the formulation models. Acknowledging points of consensus should make this discussion somewhat easier. Although there appears to be agreement among orientations about the importance of different levels of data on a vertical hierarchy, considerable differences of opinion exist about how the data on each horizontal level should be interpreted or about how the various vertical levels should be synthesized. It is in these areas that the debate among supporters of different vertical levels and horizontal models has been most acrimonious in the past. The fact is, we do not know which model is correct, and we do not currently possess a commonly accepted meta-theory to integrate vertical and horizontal data. Although most authors seem to embrace some type of comprehensive biopsychosocial approach, there is no one true, proven methodology of data synthesis. The development, analysis, and clinical testing of alternative hypotheses for this type of integration should be a major focus of future psychiatric research.

Second, convergence of perspectives on case formulation has significant ramifications for psychiatric education programs and their trainees. For psychiatric residency programs to provide a comprehensive balanced approach requires careful attention to biological, psychological, and sociocultural content of the curriculum. An overemphasis on one particular level in a vertical hierarchy should be unacceptable as should an overemphasis on a single perspective on any horizontal level. Residents must be exposed to multiple perspectives about clinical issues. Similarly, in the absence of a single meta-theory of integration, residents should also be exposed to a number of different ideas about how to synthesize clinical data.

Third, what has been said about psychiatric education programs is also true for the continuing education of practitioners trained in one particular approach. The emerging consensus about the importance of data from multiple levels and perspectives should cause some concern for clinicians who are unidimensional in their work with patients. Hopefully they will be stimulated to broaden their perspectives and seek additional training and supervision. They may ultimately be forced to do so as peer review groups and sources of reimbursement come to expect a comprehensive approach to patient care.

Finally, and perhaps most important, the recognition of the value of multiple perspectives about clinical situations should be a source of excitement and hope to clinicians. It is true that a multidimensional approach will always be more complicated than a simple consideration of data from only one particular aspect of a patient's life. But the additional knowledge and understanding gained from a balanced evaluation also yields tremendous rewards by revealing multiple avenues of potential intervention. This is especially valuable for very difficult and complex cases that challenge the stamina and will of any clinician.

In summary, there has been considerable convergence of perspectives on case formulation in recent years. Although we still await the emergence of a single meta-theory to integrate all aspects of clinical data, the points of consensus in the existing formulation models provide an excellent foundation for continued dialogue among proponents of various points of view and considerable benefit for educators, trainees, clinicians, and patients alike.

References

Abrams EM: Beyond eclecticism. Am J Psychiatry 140:740–745, 1983

Abrams GM: Psychiatric serialism. Compr Psychiatry 22:372–378, 1981

Alonso A: The psychodynamic approach, in Outpatient Psychiatry Diagnosis and Treatment, 2nd Edition. Edited by Lazare A. Baltimore, MD, Williams & Wilkins, 1989, pp 37–58

American Psychiatric Association: Diagnostic and Statistical Manual of Mental Disorders, 3rd Edition, Revised. Washington, DC, American Psychiatric Press, 1987

Beitman BD, Golfried MR, Norcross JC: The movement toward integrating the psychotherapies: an overview. Am J Psychiatry 146:138–147, 1989

Blanck G, Blanck R: Ego Psychology II. New York, Columbia University Press, 1979

Cleghorn JM: Formulation: a pedagogic antidote to DSM-III. Compr Psychiatry 26:504–512, 1985

Doherty WJ: Challenges to integration: research and clinical issues, in Family Systems in Medicine. Edited by Ramsey LN. New York, Guilford, 1989, pp 571–582

Eisenthal S: The sociocultural approach, in Outpatient Psychiatry Diagnosis and Treatment, 2nd Edition. Edited by Lazare A. Baltimore, MD, Williams & Wilkins, 1989, pp 69–102

Engle GL: The clinical application of the biopsychosocial model. Am J Psychiatry 137:535–544, 1980

Faulkner LR, Kinzie JD, Angell R, et al: A comprehensive psychiatric formulation model. Journal of Psychiatric Education 9:189–203, 1985

Fink PJ: Response to the presidential address: is "biopsychosocial" the psychiatric shibboleth? Am J Psychiatry 145:1061–1067, 1988

Glynn SM, Mueser KT, Liberman RP: The behavioral approach, in Outpatient Psychiatry Diagnosis and Treatment, 2nd Edition. Edited by Lazare A. Baltimore, MD, Williams & Wilkins, 1989, pp 59–68

Goldsmith SR, Mandell AJ: The dynamic formulation: a critique of a psychiatric ritual. Am J Psychiatry 125:152–157, 1969

Kline S, Cameron PM: I: Formulation. Canadian Psychiatric Association Journal 23:39–42, 1978

Lazare A: A multidimensional approach to psychopathology, in Outpatient Psychiatry Diagnosis and Treatment, 2nd Edition. Edited by Lazare A. Baltimore, MD, Williams & Wilkins, 1989, pp 7–16

MacKinnon RA, Yudofsky SC: DSM-III diagnosis and the psychodynamic case formulation, in The Psychiatric Evaluation in Clinical Practice. Edited by MacKinnon RA, Yudofsky SC. Philadelphia, PA, JB Lippincott, 1986, pp 213–250

Marmor J, Woods SM: The Interface Between the Psychodynamic and Behavioral Therapies. New York, Plenum, 1980

Meyersburg HA, Post RM: An holistic developmental view of neural and psychological processes: a neurobiological-psychoanalytic integration. Br J Psychiatry 135:139–155, 1979

Molina JA: Understanding the biopsychosocial model. Int J Psychiatry Med 13:29–36, 1983–84

Perry S, Cooper AM, Michels R: The psychodynamic formulation: its purpose, structure and clinical application. Am J Psychiatry 144:543–550, 1987

Rogoff M, Lazare A: The biologic approach, in Outpatient Psychiatry Diagnosis and Treatment, 2nd Edition. Edited by Lazare A. Baltimore, MD, Williams & Wilkins, 1989, pp 17–36

Ross CA, Leichner P: Canadian and British opinion on formulation. Annals of the Royal College of Physicians and Surgeons of Canada 19:49–52, 1986

Sabelli HC, Carlson-Sabelli L: Biological priority and psychological supremacy: a new integrative paradigm derived from process theory. Am J Psychiatry 146:1541–1551, 1989

von Bertalanffy L: General Systems Theory. New York, Braziller, 1968

Walsh BW, Peterson LE: Philosophical foundations of psychological theories: the issue of synthesis. Psychotherapy 22:145–153, 1985

Wolpe J, Turkat ID: Behavioral formulation of clinical cases, in Behavioral Case Formulations. Edited by Turkat ID. New York, Harper & Row, 1988, pp 5–36

Yager J: Psychiatric eclecticism: a cognitive view. Am J Psychiatry 134:736–741, 1977

CHAPTER 7

Writing Psychiatric Case Formulations

IN PREVIOUS CHAPTERS, we addressed the "What is a formulation" question and described four different orientations. In this chapter, we address the "How does one conceptualize and write a formulation" question.

Unlike Chapters 2–5, which focused on the ideological and theoretical, this chapter is decidedly pedagogical and practical. The reader should find Chapter 8 to be equally as practical and useful.

The task of writing a psychiatric formulation involves a number of challenges for the clinician. First, it dictates that the clinician review a case in depth, summarize and organize considerable data and hypotheses, and answer the descriptive question, "What happened?" Next, it requires that the clinician analyze and synthesize the case from one or more theoretical perspectives to answer the explanatory question, "Why did it happen?" Third, it stretches the clinician's creative and pragmatic potential to answer the treatment-prognostic question, "What can be done about it and how likely will it occur?" At first, these challenges can seem so overwhelming that many clinicians refrain from formally specifying a formulation.

As formidable as the task of formulation appears, it is our conviction that formulating a case is an eminently learnable and teachable skill. Like other skills, it is learned through both practice and modeling. In this chapter, we describe two formats for practicing the skills of written case formulation. In Chapter 8, we provide a number of expertly crafted written case formulations that can serve as models for the reader.

Because the biopsychosocial paradigm has been proclaimed the dominant or reigning paradigm in American psychiatry today (Fink 1988), we have chosen to highlight biopsychosocial formulations in this and the following chapter. The two different learning formats described in this chapter are those that we have developed for use in psychiatry residency education as well as for use in continuing medical education seminars. They first emerged in the course of teaching the formulation process to beginning psychiatry residents. Both formats have served as cognitive maps that residents have successfully utilized to learn the skills of case formulation. These two formats, particularly the second, can be likened to training wheels, providing considerable support while one learns the skill of riding a bike. The learner relies on the training wheels until some proficiency with the skill is achieved, and then the training wheels are no longer needed. Both of the formats presented in this chapter not only guide and influence the process of conceptualizing the formulation, but also profoundly influence the process of interviewing and data collection. Residents using these formats quickly began to think more in terms of hypotheses—data generation and collection—than in terms of the "laundry-list" approach to data gathering. Chapter 8 provides an alternative format that more experienced clinicians seem to prefer.

Format 1 for Writing Case Formulations

This format is briefer, more thematic, and more freewheeling and seems to be preferred by more visually oriented clinicians than the second format. A number of other visually represented formats have been described in the clinical literature (Leigh and Reiser 1980; Molina 1982, 1983–84; Norcombe and Gallagner 1986; Rosse 1984). Leigh and Reiser's patient evaluation grid is the most widely known. These visually represented formats are particularly useful in clarifying the interrelations of symptoms to vulnerabilities. Thus these formats are quite useful in developing the explanatory component of a formulation. Format 1, probably the easiest of the formats to learn and use, leads the clinician in a step-by-step manner from schematic representation to written report.

This format is based on seven dimensions for articulating and explaining the nature and origins of the patient's presentation and subsequent treatment. The seven dimensions will be described in terms of seven Ps: presentation, predisposition, precipitants, pattern, perpetuants, (treatment) plan, and prognosis. Table 7–1 compares the seven Ps to the three components of a psychiatric formulation.

Presentation refers to a description of nature and severity of the individual's psychiatric presentation. It can include symptoms, past history, and course of the illness. Presentation is similar to the descriptive formulation component described in Chapter 1. As such, it lends itself to being specified in DSM-III-R (American Psychiatric Association 1987) diagnostic language.

The following four Ps—predisposition, precipitants, pattern, and perpetuants—correspond to the explanatory component of a psychiatric formulation described in Chapter 1.

Predisposition refers to all factors that render an individual vulnerable to a disorder. Predisposing factors usually involve physical, psychological, and social factors. Physical or biological factors include genetic, familial, temperament, or medical patterns, such as family history of a major psychiatric disorder, an organ inferiority, family history of substance abuse, a difficult or slow-to-warm-up child temperament, or cardiac disease or hypertension. Psychological factors might include dysfunctional beliefs or convictions involving inadequacy, perfectionism, or overdependence, which might further predispose the individual to a medical disorder, such as coronary artery disease. Psychological factors might involve limited or exaggerated social skills like lack of friendship skills, unassertiveness, or overaggressiveness. Social factors could include early childhood losses, inconsistent parenting style, overly enmeshed or disengaged family of origin, or a family constellation characterized by dogged competitiveness or emotional surveillance. Subcultural, financial, and ethnic factors can be additional social predisposers.

Precipitants refer to physical, psychological, and social stressors that may be causative or coincide with the onset of symptoms or a disorder. These may include physical stressors like trauma, pain, medication side effects, or withdrawal from an addictive substance. Common psychological stressors involve losses, rejections, or disappointments that undermine a sense of personal competence. Social stressors also may involve losses or rejections that undermine an individual's social support and status. Included are illness, death, or hospitalization of a significant other, job demotion, loss of Social Security disability payments, and so on.

Table 7–1. **Comparison of the components of a psychiatric formulation with the seven Ps**

Psychiatric formulation components	P dimensions
Descriptive	Presentation
Explanatory	Predisposition
	Precipitant
	Pattern
	Perpetuants
Plan of treatment—prognostic	Plan (treatment)
	Prognosis

Pattern refers to the predictable and consistent style or manner in which a person thinks, feels, acts, copes, and defends the self both in stressful and nonstressful circumstances. It reflects the individual's baseline functioning. This pattern has physical, psychological, and social features, such as a sedentary and coronary-prone life-style, dependent personality style or disorder, or collusion in a relative's marital problems. Pattern also includes the individual's functional strengths, which counterbalance dysfunction. One way of specifying pattern is with DSM-III-R Axis II personality traits or disorder language.

Perpetuants refer to processes by which an individual's pattern is reinforced and confirmed by both the individual and the individual's environment. These processes may be physical, such as impaired immunity or habituation to an addictive substance; psychological, such as losing hope or fearing the consequences of getting well; or social, such as colluding family members or agencies that foster constrained dysfunctional behavior rather than recovery and growth.

Sometimes precipitating factors continue and become perpetuants. Precipitants and perpetuants can be recurrent or persistent, multiple or singular, cumulative or episodic. Patterns have traditionally been the focus of instrumentation in psychological assessment and the basis for a comprehensive psychiatric interview. Clinicians who can effectively elicit and articulate information on pattern as it is distinct but complementary to predisposition, precipitants, and perpetuants are cognitively aided in both case formulation and treatment planning.

Plan refers to a planned treatment intervention, including treatment goal(s), strategy, and methods. It corresponds to the first part of the "treatment-prognostic" component of a psychiatric formulation, as described in Chapter 1.

Prognosis refers to the individual's expected response to treatment. This forecast is based on the individual's strengths, premorbid pattern and level of functioning, perpetuants, capacity for treatment, expectations and motivation for treatment, and the natural history of the psychiatric disorder. Level of functioning refers to the extent to which an individual meets the challenges and tasks of life. The Global Assessment of Functioning (GAF) Scale, as used on Axis V of DSM-III-R, quantifies the individual's functioning at the time treatment is sought. In addition, it quantifies the individual's best level of functioning in the previous 12 months. Clinicians routinely assess GAF serially over the course of treatment as a change measure. The individual's capacity for treatment refers not only to degree of psychological mindedness, but also a prediction of likely change based on previous successes in life, such as with relations, job tenure, or habit change (e.g., permanent weight loss, smoking cessation). It is also based on insight and changes derived from previous therapies. Treatment capacity also includes the extent and degree of the individual's support systems, which can further reinforce and support therapy processes and outcomes. Furthermore, treatment capacity is assessed in terms of the severity and focality of symptoms. Clinical lore suggests that the more acute and focused the symptom(s), the more likely and quickly the individual will respond to treatment. On the other hand, the more chronic and diffuse the symptoms, the slower and more guarded will be the response to treatment.

Eliciting the individual's explanation for his or her symptoms or disorder—the patient's formulation—and the individual's initiation, expectations for nature, and duration of treatment further clarify the individual's likely response to the proposed, negotiated treatment plan and intervention. Finally, prognostic forecasting must include some recognition of the natural history or pathogenesis of the disorder. For instance, early and adequately treated anxiety disorders and episodes of affective disorders have a higher "cure" rate than nontreated or partially treated disorders. Specifically, untreated or partially treated panic disorders can progress to agoraphobia, or generalized anxiety disorder, to somatoform disorders, and finally to dysthymia or major depression in a matter of a few years. Cyclic pathologies such as bipolar disorder (formerly called manic depression) tend to have a waxing and waning course. Knowledge of the natural course and of how previous treatments have attenuated that course is essential to articulating an accurate clinical prognosis.

Developing and Writing the Psychiatric Formulation Summary Statement

Five components of the case formulation have been described. Developing a case formulation summary involves three steps: focused data collection, thematic configuration, and articulation of the written summary.

Focused data collection. A useful and productive clinical evaluation will elicit relevant biological, psychological, and social dimensions of pattern, predisposition, precipitants, and perpetuants as well as presentation, plan of treatment, and prognosis. As noted previously, psychiatric evaluations have typically focused on presentation, pattern, and precipitant and less on predispositions and perpetuants. To develop an integrative formulation, sufficient information on all seven Ps must be elicited and collected.

Thematic configuration. Developing a thematic configuration involves an ordering of data on presentation, predisposition, pattern, precipitants, perpetuants, plan, and prognosis. We have found the thematic chart presented in Table 7–2 to be useful in arranging case data.

The written summary. After case data have been collected and thematically related, the final step is a written articulation of the thematic schema. The written summary formulation includes seven sequential statements and is approximately 100–250 words in length. First, the patient's

Table 7–2. **Thematic configuration chart for developing formulations**

Presentation:

Bio __________ **Psych** __________ **Social** __________ **Predisposition**	**Bio** __________ **Psych** __________ **Social** __________ **Strengths** __________ **Pattern**
Precipitants 1. __________ n. __________	**Perpetuants** 1. __________ n. __________

Plan (of treatment) and prognosis:

symptom presentation is reported. Second, physical predispositions, if any, are reported, followed by psychological and social predisposers that contribute to the presenting problem(s). Third, the individual's pattern and level of functioning are described in all three spheres, if germane. Fourth, a statement of pertinent perpetuants is provided. Fifth, precipitants that have triggered or appeared concurrently with the onset of symptoms or concerns are stated. Sixth, a treatment plan is specified. Finally, a prognostic statement including the manner in which the individual appeared for treatment, as well as history and previous course of treatment of the disorder, is given.

The following case example will be used to illustrate this process of conceptualizing and writing a summary formulation statement.

The Case of Mrs. D

Mrs. D is a 32-year-old technical writer who has become increasingly panicked, depressed, and suicidal since her husband announced he was in love with another woman and was filing for divorce. Since then, she has been living alone and acknowledges insomnia, agitation, loss of appetite, difficulty concentrating, fatigue, and loss of interest in her hobbies (i.e., knitting and watching television). Mrs. D is a shy, isolated person with only one close friend and very limited emotional supports other than her husband of 5 years. Although childless, she reports that she and her husband were reasonably happy for the first 3 years of marriage. Mrs. D depended totally on her husband and seemed more concerned about losing his support than about the dissolution of the marriage. Since then, she has been experiencing episodes of panic two to three times a week. She has no prior psychiatric history, but her maternal aunt to whom she was very close had committed suicide following a long bout of depression. Mrs. D reports that she continues to be saddened when she thinks of her aunt. Mrs. D had been prescribed propranolol (Inderal) by her family doctor for the panic symptoms, which were thought to be in part related to mitral valve prolapse. She recalls being told by her parents that she was timid, frightened, and colicky as a young child.

Mrs. D describes herself as hard working, conservative, and relatively unable to express affection. She acknowledges trying to be perfect, needing to be in control of every social situation, and having an excessive commitment to work. She graduated from college with a degree in journalism while working for a government agency. Until recently, she found her job satisfying and was regularly rewarded with salary increases because of her diligence and loyalty. Mrs. D describes her family of origin as emotionally distant and detached. Although her parents were relatively well to do, she received little emotional support for pursuing outside relationships or interests. Since graduating from college, she visits her parents twice a year during holidays. Her dating history was minimal. She went out with only two men since high school and married the third during her last year of college shortly after meeting him. He became her major source of emotional support. She reports her husband had been dissatisfied with their deteriorating sexual relationship. Were it not for her panic attacks in which she becomes totally dependent on him, she believes they would still be together.

Mrs. D views herself as responsible, competent, and righteous in her work, but inadequate and fragile in social relationships. She views life as unpredictable and demanding, while insisting that someone needs to care for her needs, because she herself is unable. Subsequently, she attempts to be in control, right and proper in all situations, but emotionally clinging and feeling avoiding with selective individuals, particularly her husband. Mrs. D is not particularly psychologically minded, nor curious about inner dynamics. On the other hand, she has been relatively successful in school and on the job. She admits that she lacks self-sufficiency and that her continued overdependence on her husband was unhealthy. She is willing to work in both individual and marital therapy, even if her husband insists on divorce.

Mrs. D was adjudged a good candidate for antidepressant medication for both depressive and panic features given the biological loading for these symptoms and the fact that these represent a single episode. Psychotherapy was also recommended to focus on characterological features, which further predisposed her to depression and panic, and on couples issues, which likely reinforced her dependency and compulsivity.

Formulation summary statement: the case of Mrs. D. The following is a written formulation statement for the case of Mrs. D. Note that the seven Ps are indicated in parentheses. Table 7–3 depicts the organizing schemata for this case.

Mrs. D is a 32-year-old female, recently separated from her husband and experiencing panic attacks, suicidal ideation, and mood instability (presentation). She appears to be biologically predisposed to a major depressive episode and panic disorder. These facts coupled with her dysfunctional beliefs about perfection, clinging, and isolation and her emotionally distant and demanding family of origin (predisposition) have resulted in the development of rigid, clinging compulsive-dependent personality styles with limited coping capacity. Although occupationally adaptive and successful, this style limits efforts to relate emotionally with her husband and form

Table 7–3. **Organizing schemata for case formulation: Case of Mrs. D**

Presentation: panic attacks, suicidal ideation, and mood instability

Predisposition	Pattern
Bio Family history of depression and suicide • History of mitral valve prolapse and other possible predisposers to panic • Slow to warm up temperament as young child	**Bio** Depressive features with suicidal ideation • Panic symptoms
Psych Dysfunctional beliefs: perfectionism; feeling avoidance; social isolation/clinging	**Psych** Possible unresolved grief reaction (Aunt) • Obsessive-compulsive and dependent pattern • Limited interpersonal and coping skills • Feeling avoidance, perfectionism
Social Emotionally distant parents; possible overreliance on maternal aunt • High expectations for achievement/self-sufficiency • Few childhood friends/interests	**Social** Overdependence on husband—marital discord • Isolative; limited support system
	Strengths Occupationally adaptive and successful

Precipitants	Perpetuants
1. Physical separation from husband; loss of his emotional support	1. Husband's reinforcement of her clinging and reconfirmation of beliefs about dependency 2. Reconfirmation of her beliefs about perfectionism and feeling avoidance at home and office
Plan (of treatment) and prognosis:	Antidepressant treatment; psychotherapy for character features and couples issues; fair to good prognosis

supportive relationships (precipitants). This pattern of clinging dependency appears to have been reinforced by her husband, and her beliefs about perfectionism and feeling avoidance have probably been reinforced and reaffirmed by her employer, who rewarded accuracy and meticulousness (pattern). Subsequently, when her husband told her of his wish for a divorce, Mrs. D experienced increased panic attacks, further depression, and feelings of hopelessness and helplessness, culminating in suicidal ideation (perpetuants).

Because of the biological loading for this first episode of depression and panic, Mrs. D is a good candidate for medication and supportive care (plan). The prognosis for amelioration of panic and depressive features is good, although the prognosis for changes in her long-standing dependency and compulsivity is more guarded and depends, in large part, on her willingness to engage in longer-term therapy. The fate of her marriage depends on her willingness and the willingness of her husband to deal with their relational and sexual issues, probably in couples therapy. Her expectations for treatment are realistic, and her motivation appears sufficient. Mrs. D was able to recognize and accept that her recovery would be dependent primarily on becoming more self-sufficient (prognosis).

The DSM-III-R multiaxial diagnosis is as follows:

Axis I Major depression, single episode (296.22); panic disorder without agoraphobia, severe (300.22)
Axis II Obsessive-compulsive personality disorder (301.40); dependent personality disorder (301.60)
Axis III Mitral valve prolapse by history
Axis IV Severity of Psychosocial Stressors: 3, with moderate stress due to marital separation
Axis V Current GAF score: 40; highest GAF score past year: 68

Format 2 for Writing Case Formulations

Format 2 is more specific, structured, and systematic than Format 1. Because it is more systematic and less thematic than Format 1, it is preferred by beginning psychiatry residents. The format is based around four worksheets: descriptive-diagnostic component worksheet, explanatory component worksheet, treatment-prognostic component worksheet, and a psychiatric formulation summary worksheet (Appendix B, Worksheets 1–4). Each of these will be described briefly and illustrated with a case example. The first three worksheets focus on organizing the analysis and synthesis of case information such that the clinician can systematically generate a complete formulation that gets summarized on the psychiatric formulation sheet. This summary sheet can then be transferred, or appended, to a traditional psychiatric evaluation report.

Descriptive-Diagnostic Component Worksheet

This worksheet summarizes data in five areas: chief complaint, history of past treatment, problem list, DSM-III-R diagnosis, and prognostic index/capacity for treatment. In the problem list section, we suggest that the clinician think of short-term symptoms, behaviors, or issues as those that are acute, noncharacterological, or fairly circumscribed or that may be time limited. Furthermore, these should reflect presenting symptoms, behaviors, or issues that can be framed as "treatable" in a relatively short time. Long term refers to less focal, more characterological skills deficits, or chronic symptoms, behaviors, or issues. From a biopsychosocial perspective, the clinician may want to categorize these in terms of biological (B), psychosocial (P), or social-interpersonal-environmental (S).

A multiaxial diagnostic formulation using DSM-III-R categories is next specified. Note the space to list more than one diagnosis for Axes I and II as well as traits and/or defenses for Axis II if criteria for a specific personality disorder(s) cannot be met. Axis IV is specified by listing the principal stressor(s).

Since an Axis I diagnostic category is the least likely to suggest an effective treatment formulation and intervention—research suggests that nondiagnostic patient variables are more likely to specify effective treatment formulations and intervention (Fink 1988)—data on "capacity for treatment" are emphasized in this format. Table 7–4 lists and defines 10 such indicators of capacity for treatment. On Worksheet 1, the clinician is asked to rate these 10 indicators on these 5-point scales. Some of these indicators are widely known, such as psychological mindedness, past treatment compliance, and motivation for present treatment. After completing these ratings, the clinician looks for a pattern to the ratings. Generally speaking, the more the ratings aggregate to the right, the more likely the patient will be amenable to treatment that is shorter, more focused, and more responsive to insight or dynamically oriented therapies, while at the same time suggesting a more positive prognosis. On the other hand, ratings that aggregate more to the left margin suggest that treatment will be complex, less likely to be responsive to dynamic and insight-oriented methods, with a more guarded prognosis.

Explanatory Component Worksheet

This worksheet requires the clinician to analyze, synthesize, and summarize data in terms of the five Ps of precipitant, pattern, perpetuant, predisposition, and prognosis. These terms were defined and illustrated earlier.

Here, pattern, predisposition, and perpetuants are specified in terms of the biological, psychological, and social-interpersonal-systematic domains. Key terms and concepts are provided to facilitate the clinician's thinking. The clinician is asked to translate the ratings on prognosis and patient capacity from the descriptive-diagnostic worksheet to narrative form on this worksheet. Table 7– 4 offers operational definitions for terms relating to the patient's capacity for treatment.

Table 7– 4. **Guide to terminology in evaluating a patient's capacity for psychiatric treatment**

defensive style a measure of the patient's method of coping with internal and external conflict. The patient with the rejecting style will project blame and displace conflict outwardly through acting out and/or somatization. Patients with more accepting styles channel conflict more through emotion and use less primitive defenses, and thus are more appropriate for insight and dynamic therapies.

explanatory style a measure of locus of control or how the patient explains his or her problems/symptoms by attributing them to either "external" causes and thus rejecting or minimizing personal responsibility or "internal" causes by which personal responsibility is recognized and accepted.

information style preferred style or means of processing session information through visual (V), auditory (A), or kinesthetic (K) channels. Research indicates that patients with visual-auditory (A or VA) styles relate better to dynamic-insight therapies than patients with kinesthetic styles, who relate better to action-oriented therapies.

motivation for present treatment a measure of the likelihood that a patient will remain in treatment and profit from it. Patients with high motivation are likely to be self-referred, want to change, have ego-dystonic symptoms, and have had positive "change" experiences in their lives, as compared with patients with low motivation, who are referred to treatment by others, have little desire to change, have symptoms that are ego-synteric, and have few if any positive change experiences in their lives.

past treatment compliance a predictive measure of the likelihood the patient will adhere to the present treatment. In reviewing the patient's compliance history, assess the degree of compliance with medications, appointments, therapeutic involvement, intersession assignments, and so on. Past noncompliance usually predicts the present level of compliance.

psychological mindedness a measure of both the patient's capacity and motivation for introspection and ability to recognize the influence of the past on the present and to communicate thoughts, feelings, and fantasies. High levels of this measure are correlated positively with response to dynamic therapies.

Table 7–4. **Continued**

reactance a measure of the patient's persuasibility or compliance with external demands. The higher the patient's level of reactance, the higher the degree to which the patient will be receptive to therapeutic interventions (e.g., interpretive). Lower reactance suggests more opposition and resistance to the therapist's influence; thus, the indication for the use of therapeutic paradox and "waiting for change" to occur are important.

social support system a measure of the extent of consistent personal and institutional ties that serve to "buffer" the patient from stressors and increase sense of self-cohesiveness and life's meaning. "Weaker" social supports and the inconsistency and/or overintrusiveness of these supports are correlated with increased recidivism, medication and treatment noncompliance, and suicidality.

symptom focality a measure of symptom complexity ranging from high or monosymptomatic (e.g., public-speaking phobias in an otherwise high-functioning person) to low multisymptomatic (e.g., a person with borderline personality with chronic anxious, dysphoric, and dissociative features).

symptom severity a measure of symptom disruption in the patient's life. The more life tasks involved (e.g., work, school, family, friends), the greater the severity. The higher the Global Assessment of Functioning Scale score, the more "mild" and likely the patient can respond to dynamic therapies.

Treatment-Prognostic Component Worksheet

While the other worksheets rely on the clinician's abilities to think convergently and deductively, this worksheet requires the abilities to think more divergently and inductively. The patient's expectations of treatment are specified as are treatment goals and outcomes. Goal specification should parallel the problem specification on the descriptive-diagnostic worksheet. In other words, if "social isolation and limited relational skills" are specified as a basic problem, "increased socialization and relational skills" can be specified as treatment goals. Treatment goals are sometimes described as either process or outcome goals. Process goals usually refer to intermediate goals that can be advised during the process of treatment, such as increases in engagement treatment and self-exploration. Outcome goals refer to outcomes apparent outside treatment, such as "amelioration of panic symptoms."

The section on rationale for treatment plan decisions requires some explanation. The challenge of prescribing effective, efficient treatment is to define clearly what works best for whom and in what setting and time frame. Differential therapeutics is the name given to this endeavor to tailor or match treatment to patient needs, expectations, and style (Frances et al. 1984; Perry et al. 1985). Advocates of differential therapeutics like Frances et al. (1984) believe that all forms of psychiatric treatment have five inherent axes that need to be considered in treatment selection: setting, format, duration and frequency, treatment modality, and the need for somatic treatment. Setting refers to where treatment occurs: in a clinic, inpatient unit, day hospital, or halfway house. Format is determined by who directly participates in the treatment: individual, marital, family, or group. Time refers to both the length of each session and the frequency of the sessions. Treatment modality refers to the range of psychosocial interventions. Somatic treatments include medications, electroconvulsive therapy, dietary change, psychosurgery, and so on. In addition, a metadecision that overrides the consideration of each of these five components must be addressed. This is a consideration of "no treatment" as the prescription of choice. Clinicians are asked not only to indicate their treatment decision in each of the areas, but to specify their reasons or rationale for their choice.

The Case of R.F.

R.F. is a 32-year-old, single, white male seen on consultation with complaints of fatigue and dysphoria of several years' duration, as well as a number of somatic symptoms, the most distressing of which is awakening from sleep in a panic gasping for air. This symptom of recent onset had become progressively worse in the past 4 days, prompting this consultation.

He reports a long history of psychiatric treatment since the age of 15, last being hospitalized 5 years ago for a psychotic episode following binge drinking. He reported a "blasphemous dream in which I thought I cursed Christ and began to fear going to sleep." R.F. believes this dream meant that he was damned if he did not remain vigilant and awake at night. His fatigue symptoms and dysphoria date from this event, 8 months ago from an overdose of perphenazine-amitriptyline (Triavil) following an altercation with his father about continuing to live in the family home. After discharge he was treated in a day hospital program for 3 months before dropping out due to being "too fatigued to stay awake in groups all day." Since then he has been followed for monthly medication checks at a community mental health clinic. R.F. was relatively compliant with amitriptyline (Elavil) 250 mg for 4 months after hospitalization despite complaints of dry mouth and fatigue. In the month prior to this evaluation, he had been switched to doxepin (Sinequan) 150 mg—with trace serum levels and the onset of the apnea-like symptoms.

R.F.'s family history is positive for heart disease, diabetes, and hypertension, with a maternal uncle in a state hospital with chronic undifferentiated schizophrenia and a maternal grandfather in end-stage Alzheimer's disease. No drug or alcohol abuse is noted in the family, except for the patient's own occasional binge-drinking episodes. He denies any major medical problems, although he has gained 40 pounds and reports he snores loudly and experiences myoclonic leg movements. His diet appears poorly balanced, and he gets little or no exercise.

He is the younger of two siblings; his sister is 4 years older and married to a carpenter. His father is described as being demanding and critical and as having been browbeaten by his own father (the patient's grandfather) because R.F. has no job and continues to live at home. R.F.'s mother is described as being overly protective and appears to infantilize R.F. The marital relationship is described as alternating between being distant and being conflictual. It appears that the patient's function is as a foil and peacemaker for his parents' interaction. R.F. completed high school with barely passing grades, never dated, and was teased by peers of being gay, which he denies. He has had no regular friends for nearly 5 years and experiences little concern in forming or maintaining friendships. He has worked in several blue-collar jobs in the service industry, the last job as a baker. He typically quit or was fired from a job for lack of interest or for excessive absences after 3 or 4 months. Presently, he lives at home with both parents since losing his last job 3 years ago, but is becoming increasingly pressured by his father to become financially independent since his father is soon to retire.

The mental status examination showed a moderately obese, adequately groomed, right-handed, expressionless man who was fully oriented to four spheres with somewhat of a whiny speech of normal rate and prosody that was goal directed. Affect was constricted, with mild to moderate dysphoric mood. His presentation was unremarkable for psychotic features and homicidal, suicidal, or paranoid ideation. Although he admitted being extremely anxious, there was no obvious sign of discomfort in his manner or voice. Insight was limited, and judgment was mildly impaired.

R.F. believes his condition is caused by fatigue and that his fatigue is secondary to his fear of falling asleep. His expectation of treatment is symptom relief only. He is willing to take medication but is reluctant to have "any more talking therapy." However, he agrees to a behavioral approach. Past compliance has been poor when secondary gain issues were involved, but with relatively good compliance with medication.

Formulation of the Case of R.F.: Worksheets. The case of R.F. is presented in Appendix B, Worksheets 5–8. The reader will note that Worksheet 8 is a summary statement of the data/hypotheses specified on Worksheets 5–7. The contents of the worksheet could be then transferred to traditional case report formats and/or become part of the patient's permanent chart.

References

American Psychiatric Association: Diagnostic and Statistical Manual of Mental Disorders, 3rd Edition, Revised. Washington, DC, American Psychiatric Association, 1987

Fink P: Response to the presidential address: is "biopsychosocial" the psychiatric shibboleth? Am J Psychiatry 145:1061–1067, 1988

Frances A, Clarkin J, Perry S: Differential Therapeutics in Psychiatry: The Art and Science of Treatment Selection. New York, Brunner/Mazel, 1984

Leigh H, Reiser MF: The Patient: Biological, Psychological and Social Dimension of Medical Practice. New York, Plenum, 1980

Molina JA: Psychobiosocial "maps": a useful tool in milieu and psychiatric education. J Clin Psychiatry 43:182–186, 1982

Molina JA: Understanding the biopsychosocial model. Int J Psychiatry Med 13:29–35, 1983–84

Norcombe B, Gallagner RM: The Clinical Process in Psychiatry: Diagnosis and Management Planning. Cambridge, England, Cambridge University Press, 1986

Perry S, Frances A, Clarkin J: A DSM-III Casebook of Differential Therapeutics. New York, Brunner/Mazel, 1985

Rosse RB: Biopsychosocial "mapping" with medical students in consultation-liaison psychiatry. Int J Psychiatry Med 14:323–330, 1984

Appendix B

Worksheets That Form the Basis for Writing Case Formulations

Worksheet 1. **Descriptive-diagnostic component worksheet**

Patient's name ________________ Age _____ Case no. ____________
Date of intake ________________
Chief complaint ____

History of past treatment ____________________________________
____
____
____

Problem list

Short term	Long term
________________	________________
________________	________________
________________	________________
________________	________________
________________	________________
________________	________________

Differential diagnostic formulation

Axis I ____
____
R/O ____
Axis II ____
____
(traits/defenses) ____________________________________
Axis III ____
____
R/O ____
Axis IV stressors: family/job/loss/finances/other ______________
____
Severity ____
Axis V GAF now ______________ Highest in 12 mo ______________

Prognostic index/capacity for treatment (place an *X* or code)

1.	Symptom severity	severe	├──┼──┼──┼──┤	mild
2.	Symptom focality	low	├──┼──┼──┼──┤	high
3.	Defensive style	reject	├──┼──┼──┼──┤	accept
4.	Social support system	weak	├──┼──┼──┼──┤	strong
5.	Psychological mindedness	low	├──┼──┼──┼──┤	high
6.	Explanatory style	external	├──┼──┼──┼──┤	internal
7.	Past Tx compliance	low	├──┼──┼──┼──┤	high
8.	Past Tx compliance (therapy)	low	├──┼──┼──┼──┤	high
9.	Motivation for present Tx	low	├──┼──┼──┼──┤	high
10.	Information style	kinesthetic	├──┼──┼──┼──┤	auditory

Prognosis ____
____
____

Note. R/O = rule out. GAF = Global Assessment of Functioning Scale. Tx = treatment.

Worksheet 2. **Explanatory component worksheet**

Patient's name ________________ Age ____ Case no. __________

P1

Precipitating event(s) ____

____

____

____

P2–4: Pattern/Perpetuants/Predisposition

Biological: family Hx/medical Hx/health behaviors/AODA Hx

____

____

____

____

____

____

Psychological: personality dynamics; conflict & defense mechanisms/ dysfunctional cognitions & skills deficits

____

____

____

____

____

____

Social/interpersonal/systemic: role in family of origin/demands/support of job, friends, spouse, family, etc.

____

____

____

____

____

____

P5: *Patient capacity for Tx* (see Descriptive-Diagnostic Formulation)

____

____

____

____

P6: *Prognosis* ____

____

____

____

Note. Hx = history. AODA = alcohol or drug abuse. Tx = treatment.

Worksheet 3. **Treatment-prognostic component worksheet**

Patient's name ________________ Age _____ Case no. ____________

Patient's expectations for current treatment

Expected Tx outcome	Patient's expected Tx method
___ Sx relief only	___ Rx only
___ Interpersonal resolution	___ Therapy only: support/ insight/action
___ Character change	___ Rx plus therapy
___ Other________________	___ Other____________

Treatment outcome goals

	Short term	Long term
Bio	____________________	____________________
	____________________	____________________
Psy	____________________	____________________
	____________________	____________________
Soc	____________________	____________________
	____________________	____________________

Rationale for treatment plan decisions (circle)

1. *Setting:* crisis — outpatient only — outpatient & day hospital — other (list) ______________________________

____

2. *Format:* individual — group therapy — Rx group — marital/family — Rx monitoring — combined treatment — other (list)

____

____

3. *Duration:* short term with termination date — short term — longer term

____

____

4. *Frequency:* 1/week — 2/month — 1/month — other (list) ________

____

____

5. *Tx strategy:* behavioral — cognitive — supportive/reality — exploratory — other (list) ______________________________

____

____

6. *Somatic Tx:* antidepressant — neuroleptic — anxiolytic — other (list)

____

____

Note. Tx = treatment. Sx = symptoms. Rx = prescription.

Worksheet 4. **Psychiatric formulation summary sheet**

Psychiatric formulation summary sheet for ______________________
(patient's name & case no.)

Descriptive-diagnostic formulation ______________________

DSM-III-R
Axis I. ______________________
Axis II. ______________________
Axis III. ______________________
Axis IV. ______________ Severity ________
Axis V. Current GAF ______ Highest GAF in 12 mo ________

Etiologic formulation: Notate each of the six parts of the formulation by the appropriate number: 1) predisposition 2) precipitant 3) pattern 4) perpetuant 5) capacity for treatment 6) prognosis

Treatment formulation

A. Treatment goals ______________________

B. Treatment approach
1. Setting ______________________
2. Mode ______________________
3. Duration ______________________
4. Strategies/methods ______________________
5. Rx ______________________

Note. GAF = Global Assessment of Functioning Scale. Rx = prescription.

Worksheet 5. **Descriptive-diagnostic component worksheet for R.F.**

Patient's name R.F. Age 32 Case no. 318-02-4621
Date of intake ____________

Chief complaint Sleep apnea-like Sx; fatigue and dysphoria

History of past treatment single, white male with continuous psychiatric Tx × 4 yr w/ 2 hospitalizations, but poor treatment compliance. Dropped out of day treatment 5 months ago, now monthly Rx monitoring: Elavil to 250 mg then switch to Sinequan to 150 mg when apnea reported.

Problem list

Short term	Long term
Sleep apnea-like Sx with dysphoria	Obesity & passive-aggressive
	Somatizing style
Tx noncompliance	Separation-individuation issues
Limited coping; assertiveness	Alexithymia
Isolative life-style & rejection-sensitivity	Occupational problems
	Family enmeshment

Differential diagnostic formulation

Axis I dysthymia; somatoform disorder NOS (300.70), hypersomnia disorder (780.50)

R/O delusional disorder—persecutory type

Axis II personality disorder NOS (avoidant, passive-aggressive, paranoid traits) (301.9)

(traits/defenses) denial

Axis III sleep apnea

R/O central vs. drug induced

Axis IV stressors: family/job/loss/finances/other no friends, no job, prospects; father's ultimatum to leave home

Severity 3–4 moderate

Axis V GAF now 45 Highest in 12 mo 52

Prognostic index/capacity for treatment (place an *X* or code*)

			Rating	
1.	Symptom severity	severe	X at 2nd of 5	mild
2.	Symptom focality	low	B at 2nd, S at 5th	high
3.	Defensive style	reject	X at 2nd	accept
4.	Social support system	weak	X at 2nd	strong
5.	Psychological mindedness	low	X at 3rd	high
6.	Explanatory style	external	X at 3rd	internal
7.	Past Tx compliance	low	X at 2nd	high
8.	Past Tx compliance (therapy)	low	A at 2nd, R at 4th	high
9.	Motivation for present Tx	low	B at 2nd, S at 5th	high
10.	Information style	kinesthetic	X at 3rd	auditory

Prognosis Fair to good for Sx relief and compliance with short-term Tx issues; at present it appears that prognosis is very guarded for long-term Tx issues

Note. Sx = symptoms. Tx = treatment. Rx = prescription. NOS = not otherwise specified. R/O = rule out. GAF = Global Assessment of Functioning Scale.

*A = scheduled appointments. B = behavior. R = medication. S = sleep.

Worksheet 6. **Explanatory component worksheet for R.F.**

Patient's name R.F. Age 32 Case no. 318-02-4621

P1

Precipitating event(s) Recent switch to Sinequan; father's ultimatum to move out of the house

P2–4: Pattern/Perpetuants/Predisposition

Biological: family Hx/medical Hx/health behaviors/AODA Hx
Sensitivity to amphetamines, sedating tricyclics, and alcohol; morbid obesity; sedentary life-style; binge-drinking Hx

Psychological: personality dynamics; conflict & defense mechanisms/ dysfunctional cognitions & skills deficits
Inactive; isolative style and extreme dependence on parents; deficits in assertiveness, feeling expression, and negotiation skills; views self as inadequate but entitled; denial

Social/interpersonal/systemic: role in family of origin/demands/support of job, friends, spouse, family, etc.
Enmeshed family network that reinforces his abnormal illness behavior and neutralizes parental demands and maternal overprotectiveness, noncompliance as system balancing

P5: *Patient capacity for Tx* (see Descriptive-Diagnostic Formulation)
Past history of minimal Tx involvement in psychosocial issues; appears receptive to work on short-term issues, especially if the treatment is Sx-oriented or behavior-oriented, but not long-term issues

P6: *Prognosis* Good for Sx relief/short term; very guarded for long-term issues

Note. Hx = history. AODA = alcohol or drug abuse. Tx = treatment. Sx = symptoms.

Worksheet 7. **Treatment-prognostic component worksheet for R.F.**

Patient's name R.F. Age 32 Case no. 318-02-4621

Patient's expectations for current treatment

Expected Tx outcome
- X Sx relief only
- ___ Interpersonal resolution
- ___ Character change
- ___ Other ___

Patient's expected Tx method
- ___ Rx only
- ___ Therapy only: support/insight/action
- ___ Rx plus therapy
- X Other Rx & behavior therapy

Treatment outcome goals

	Short term	Long term
Bio	Resolve sleep apnea	Decrease somatization; weight management
Psy	Enhance Tx compliance	Increase individuation
Soc	Increase socialization skills & behaviors	Increase occupational/ interpersonal skills

Rationale for treatment plan decisions (circle)

1. *Setting:* crisis — outpatient only — outpatient & day hospital — other (list) written contract needed; encourage day treatment as adjunctive at later time

2. *Format:* individual — group therapy — Rx goup — marital/family — Rx monitoring — combined treatment — other (list) individual sessions with at least one family evaluation session

3. *Duration:* short term with termination date — short term — longer term
eight sessions then reevaluate; schedule follow-up at 3 & 6 months

4. *Frequency:* 1/week — 2/month — 1/month — other (list) intensive treatment until sleep apnea resolves then weekly until short-term goals achieved

5. *Tx strategy:* behavioral — cognitive — supportive/reality — exploratory — other (list) sleep hygiene; sleep-activity diary; audiotape 1 night's sleep; friendship skills and time management; consider paradoxical strategies; passive-aggressive hinders Tx

6. *Somatic Tx:* antidepressant — neuroleptic — anxiolytic — other (list)
1) sleep latency studies after discontinuing Sinequan to R/O central apnea
2) protriptyline trial because of its activating properties

Note. Tx = treatment. Sx = symptoms. Rx = prescription. R/O = rule out.

Worksheet 8. **Psychiatric formulation summary sheet for R.F.**

Psychiatric formulation summary sheet for R.F. 318-02-4621
(patient's name & case no.)

Descriptive-diagnostic formulation 32-year-old obese, single, white male with sleep apnea, fatigue, and dysphoria with Hx of continuous Tx × 4 yr including 2 hospitalizations—last 8 months ago, followed by day treatment × 3 months; then on monthly Rx checks with poor compliance; Rx: Elavil to 250 mg then Sinequan to 150 mg

DSM-III-R

Axis I. dysthymia: somatoform disorder NOS; transient hypersomnia resolving

Axis II. personality disorder NOS (avoidant, passive-aggressive, paranoid traits)

Axis III. sleep apnea (medication induced)

Axis IV. family demands, no job, friends Severity 3–4 moderate

Axis V. Current GAF 45 Highest GAF in 12 mo 56

Etiologic formulation: Notate each of the six parts of the formulation by the appropriate number: 1) predisposition 2) precipitant 3) pattern 4) perpetuant 5) capacity for treatment 6) prognosis

This patient presented with 2 distinct problems, sleep apnea secondary to Sinequan in a patient exquisitely sensitive to anticholinergics, alcohol, and amphetamines. Fatigue and dysphoria appear to be a function of this patient's limited coping skills, denial, his self-perception as inadequate but entitled, and his enmeshed family of origin. He is extremely dependent on his parents, and his Sx serve to neutralize his father's high expectations and demands and his mother's overprotectiveness (1, 3). His isolative style and obesity reinforce his limited functioning in terms of friends and job (4). A recent change in Sinequan and father's ultimatum for patient to move out seem to have precipitated present crisis (2). Fair prognosis for treatment of acute problems (6) if treatment Sx-focused and behavioral in nature (5).

Treatment formulation

A. Treatment goals First, resolve sleep apnea. Then attempt to enhance treatment compliance and increase social behaviors and activities. Longer-term goals are dependent on patient's extended Tx contract.

B. Treatment approach

1. Setting outpatient, day treatment as useful adjunct but patient refuses
2. Mode individual Tx for now; later consider "shyness" group
3. Duration 3 months for skill-based Tx, then renegotiate for other issues
4. Strategies/methods explicit Tx contract with behavioral, psychoeducational, and supportive methods, because of patient's low psych mindedness, alexithymia, and expectation for treatment
5. Rx discontinue Sinequan; trial of protriptyline because of its activating properties; consider sleep latency studies if no improvement

Note. Hx = history. Tx = treatment. Rx = prescription. NOS = not otherwise specified. GAF = Global Assessment of Functioning Scale. Sx = symptoms.

CHAPTER 8

Psychiatric Case Formulations: Examples of Written Formulations

IN THIS CHAPTER, WE PRESENT four brief case histories, each of which is formulated in a biopsychosocial framework. Following each case history is a formal DSM-III-R (American Psychiatric Association 1987) diagnosis on all five axes followed by a biopsychosocial matrix that identifies the major influences (explanatory and descriptive) and interventions (treatment and prognosis) in the biological, psychological, and social domains. Following this, the formulation is given in a narrative manner. Psychological factors may include both psychodynamic and behavioral aspects, and the latter can also be found in the social domain.

Dementia Case

Mr. E is a 67-year-old retired market analyst who sold his home and moved to a retirement village after his wife's death 2 years ago. His married daughter has made an outpatient appointment for him to be seen in consultation. She is concerned that for the past 6 months her father has become increasingly forgetful and apathetic. He seems disinterested in mealtimes and on several occasions has had temper outbursts following disagreements with his bridge partners. His daughter states that her father was always an independent, strong-willed individual, the oldest of six children born to a German immigrant clock maker. She recalls that Mr. E has been reasonably fit all his life apart from a chronic peptic ulcer, which she thinks has been in remission with treatment with cimetidine. Mr. E himself agrees only grudgingly to be seen provided that "he doesn't have to take any damn fool medicines."

DSM-III-R

The DSM-III-R multiaxial diagnosis is as follows:

Axis I Primary degenerative dementia of Alzheimer type (290.13). Rule out major depression (296.20)
Axis II Rule out personality disorder with obsessional traits (301.40)
Axis III Peptic ulcer (in remission)
Axis IV Severity of Psychosocial Stressors: 3, high level of social expectation (enduring)
Axis V Current Global Assessment of Functioning (GAF) score: 40; highest GAF score past year: 90

Biopsychosocial Matrix

The biopsychosocial matrix is as follows:

	Influences (explanatory—descriptive)	**Interventions (treatment—prognosis)**
BIO	Primary degenerative dementia Rule out major depression	Dementia workup Trial of antidepressant medication
PSYCHO	High need for control Reluctance to seek support Loss of wife	Attention to compliance issues Stress self-control and autonomy
SOCIAL	High level of social expectation and demand	Move to more structured, supportive, less demanding environment Capitalize on daughter's support

Biopsychosocial Formulation

A 67-year-old man with no previous psychiatric illness presents with a 6-month history of apathy, memory loss, temper outbursts, and querulous behavior. The most likely cause is that Mr. E is developing primary degenerative dementia. Since there is no history of hypertension or stroke, the probable diagnosis is Alzheimer's disease. It is also possible that Mr. E has a major depression, and mental status examination might reveal other clinical features, such as insomnia or suicidal ideation. Further history taking from the daughter might reveal other family members who have suffered from an affective disorder. The compulsive and independent aspects of Mr. E's personality make him sensitive to the loss of control inflicted by his memory impairment, particularly in a relatively novel environment where his own expectations for social performance may be high. Although his wife's death probably is not a direct cause for any current depression, the absence of a familiar supportive figure may certainly worsen it. With the encouragement of his daughter, Mr. E should be persuaded to undergo a dementia workup to confirm the diagnosis while stressing that this may lead to interventions that will strengthen control over the situation. Physical examination should be undertaken to rule out hypertension and atherosclerosis, and mental status examination could reveal the extent of depression and memory loss. Laboratory tests should also be undertaken to confirm that his peptic ulcer is inactive and that there is no evidence of any anemia or other contributory cause for the change in mental status. A computed tomography scan and neuropsychological testing will probably confirm diffuse cortical atrophy, probable Alzheimer's dementia, and a degree of depression that is moderate to severe. Mr. E should then be persuaded to move to a less demanding and more structured and supportive environment with his daughter's encouragement and daily visits during the transitional period. Mr. E's strong belief in autonomy and refusal to accept medications would not be initially challenged. After he has settled in his new environment, antidepressant medication should be offered as an adjunct to provide restful sleep and to enhance his own ability to cope. A low dose of nortriptyline should be prescribed with plasma level monitoring. On this regimen, there will probably be a modest improvement in sleep, social interactions, and the ability to learn provided there are frequent repetitions. Mr. E's daughter would be informed that continued memory loss should be expected, with a reduction in capacity for independent living, and she should prepare for the fact that a total care facility would eventually be necessary. Once Mr. E's environment became less demanding and his depression was treated, further loss of behavioral control would be unlikely.

Delirium Case

Ms. S is a 35-year-old, pale, thin woman who lives alone and works as an executive secretary. She was admitted to the hospital for investigation of unexplained weight loss and recurrent abdominal pain. Three days after an exploratory laparotomy she became suddenly confused and disoriented and required physical restraint after she accused the nursing staff of poisoning her food and then attempted to open her abdominal wound. Ms. S's only visitor is her elderly employer, who states that this secretary is a shy, private individual whose only living relative is a father who she visits weekly in a nursing home and to whom she seems closely attached. He adds that Ms. S has always been sickly, takes frequent days off from work, and has no friends among the other secretaries, although she has worked for his company for 15 years. Apart from this, she is a conscientious, hard-working woman who seldom makes mistakes.

DSM-III-R

The DSM-III-R multiaxial diagnosis is as follows:

Axis I Delirium (293.00)
Axis II Rule out personality disorder with obsessional, avoidant features (301.90)
Axis III Diagnosis deferred (weight loss and abdominal pain), S/P laparotomy
Axis IV Severity of Psychosocial Stressors: 3, admission to hospital (acute)
Axis V Current GAF score: 30; highest GAF score past year: 70

Biopsychosocial Matrix

The biopsychosocial matrix is as follows:

	Influences (explanatory—descriptive)	**Interventions** (treatment—prognosis)
BIO	Rule out toxic, metabolic, infectious, nutritional causes Rule out sleep deprivation Rule out drug withdrawal	Laboratory investigation Consider EEG/computed tomography Consider low-dosage neuroleptic Night-light in room
PSYCHO	Loss of personal autonomy, control, and privacy	Patient involvement in decisions Prior instruction in all procedures
SOCIAL	Unaccustomed proximity to strangers Lack of familiar social support	Primary care nursing Own room (if possible)

Biopsychosocial Formulation

Ms. S is a 35-year-old single woman who has no previous psychiatric history, although she is a shy, avoidant, and mildly obsessional person with no close friends and a tendency toward somatization. Three days after an exploratory laparotomy (which revealed chronic diverticulitis and adhesions), she has developed an acute delirium, including delusions that have a paranoid and erotic content. Her frequent use of physicians in the past raises the question of possible prior substance abuse with postoperative drug withdrawal, but contact with her internist confirms that she has always been reluctant to take analgesics or tranquilizers for fear of losing control. Her employer is convinced she does not have an alcohol problem. All of the laboratory investigations proved to be normal, and a decision to investigate further for intracerebral or metabolic causes of delirium with an electroencephalogram, computed tomography scan, or lumbar puncture will be deferred until after a trial with psychotropic medication. It is noted that Ms. S has slept poorly since the operation, has appeared frightened, and has complained frequently to the nurses about having to share her room with a stranger. They also note that she became particularly agitated after her employer's most recent visit. It is probable that the delirium is secondary to sleep deprivation, itself related to stress due to loss of autonomy in an individual who has a strong need for control and privacy. A recommendation would be made to place the patient in a room of her own with a night-light, and a discussion with the nursing staff would be held to stress the importance of regular contact with a familiar nurse. In view of Ms. S's probable ambivalence toward older men, it was suggested that her employer not visit until her mental status was fully recovered, although appreciation should be expressed for his supportive intentions. The medical staff would be advised of the patient's need to be kept informed of procedures and progress and to be involved in decisions. It is highly likely that the patient's delirium will recover rapidly and completely within 24–48 hours of restoring restful sleep, with either a low-dose neuroleptic or short-acting hypnotic. This could be discontinued as soon as the patient was fully recovered.

Somatoform Pain Disorder Case

Mrs. D is a 48-year-old second-generation Polish immigrant who has had intense chronic low-back pain for 2 years and was referred for consultation as part of an evaluation for an inpatient chronic pain management program. She is accompanied to the appointment by her husband, an older man who insists on being present during the interview and who has a long list of doctors his wife has seen and medications she has taken. Mrs. D's symptoms began following a fall at work shortly after she had been promoted from assembly line worker to floor supervisor. Her husband states that she "lived for her work" and has been devastated by her inability to return following a failed lumbar laminectomy performed by a surgeon he describes as "grossly incompetent." During the interview, the patient herself expresses very little affect, although she seems close to tears at times. She claims to remember little about her childhood but her husband interrupts to explain that her father was "a mean bastard."

DSM-III-R

The DSM-III-R multiaxial diagnosis is as follows:

Axis I	Somatoform pain disorder (307.80), rule out affective disorder, rule out opioid dependence
Axis II	Rule out dependent personality disorder (301.60)
Axis III	S/P lumbar laminectomy
Axis IV	Severity of Psychosocial Stressors: 3, chronic physical discomfort
Axis V	Current GAF score: 50; highest GAF score past year: 50

Biopsychosocial Matrix

The biopsychosocial matrix is as follows:

	Influences (explanatory—descriptive)	**Interventions** (treatment—prognosis)
BIO	Lumbar disc lesion Dependency on opioid analgesics Loss of stamina/fatigue	Weaning from analgesics Initiation of tricyclic antidepressants Graduated exercise regimen
PSYCHO	Alexithymia Major depression Conflicts around dependency and aggression	Individual psychotherapy (cognitive-behavioral) Distraction procedures Relaxation training
SOCIAL	Potential litigation Reinforcement by husband Loss of work	Settlement of case Couples therapy Phased reentry

Biopsychosocial Formulation

Like most patients with somatoform pain disorder, this 48-year-old woman is enmeshed in a complex web of circumstances that sustain her condition. While she has disability disproportionate to any biomedical disease process, she certainly has physical problems secondary to her lumbar disc lesion and surgery. In addition, like a majority of chronic pain patients, history taking will also probably confirm that she has a major depression (possibly with melancholic features) and has become dependent on opiate analgesics prescribed by her orthopedic surgeon. As her pain tolerance and depression have worsened, her diminishing levels of activity have created a vicious cycle of reduced stamina and increasing fatigue. Her pain is sustained by several psychological factors. Following a physically and sexually abusive relationship with her father, she has marked conflicts around dependency issues and with the expression of aggression. Her promotion at work moved her from a lower-level position compatible with her own dependency needs to a position of authority, which aroused her own anxieties around aggression and independence. The fact that Mrs. D has restricted emotional insight and vocabulary of both cultural and familial origin prevents her from expressing and resolving this conflict and has created the primary gain for her symptoms. This resulted in leaving her job and escape from an untenable situation. Her pain behavior is also maintained by the solicitous caretaking of her husband (secondary gain or positive reinforcement), who shares her belief in an unresolved organic cause and the need for litigation. Loss of work, while resolving the anxiety and conflict of the job situation, has resulted in a substantial loss of other reinforcers and contributed to the present focus on pain and suffering. Chronic pain of such an entrenched nature would require an initial period of inpatient treatment. Following a thorough reassessment of her physical condition (to ensure confidence that nothing has been overlooked), the patient and her husband would be invited to participate in a rehabilitative program that would stress coping rather than cure. Mrs. D would be started on a low dose of a tricyclic antidepressant (with plasma level monitoring) sufficient to restore restful sleep, and she would then be weaned off her opiate analgesic. Mrs. D would begin a program of progressive muscular retraining to restore stamina and activity levels and would be given relaxation and distraction procedures to help minimize and cope with her pain. Psychotherapy would initially be cognitive and behavioral to deal with negative schemata and pain engrams, but if she showed increasing ability for emotional expression and insight, her conflicts and her early childhood experiences might be dealt with more directly at a later date.

Her husband would be invited to engage in couples therapy, with the focus around rewarding and attending to positive accomplishments and rehabilitative efforts and minimizing or ignoring pain behavior (with the patient's own understanding that talking about pain often worsens it). Both the patient and her husband would be strongly encouraged to settle any litigation at the earliest possible time. The incompatibility between attempting to reduce pain while waiting to be rewarded for it would be made clear. As soon as Mrs. D had begun to make substantial progress, a phased return to work could be negotiated with her employers for a job compatible with her physical and psychological capabilities. Like the majority of patients with chronic pain, Mrs. D is unlikely to show a complete recovery but may attain a level of functional capacity where she is able to return to some work, is no longer dependent on analgesics, and has an improved social and marital relationship that no longer focuses on pain.

Dysthymia/Double Depression Case

The utilization review coordinator of a local health maintenance organization has requested an outside opinion concerning the need for further treatment of a 43-year-old woman who has so far received 12 outpatient psychotherapy sessions without significant improvement. Mrs. C grew up in Mississippi, the youngest of 11 children born to a tenant farmer who died in a tractor accident when the patient was 6 years old. Mrs. C had vague recollections of her father as "strong and kind." Her mother worked as a hotel maid. Mrs. C was raised by older siblings, who made sure she attended school and got good grades. As soon as she graduated from high school, Mrs. C moved north to live with cousins. Soon after, she married her first husband, who was alcoholic and left her with twin daughters to raise. She married again soon after and had three more children, the youngest of whom is now 15. Throughout her adult life, Mrs. C has had "fits of the blues," often when things went wrong, but at times for no reason she could fathom. Several times she sought advice from her minister at church, but on this occasion he had suggested she obtain more formal help because of fleeting suicidal ideas. On reviewing the chart, the consultant noted that Mrs. C was being seen by an older female therapist and that the focus had been mainly on marital issues but that Mrs. C had refused several offers of couples therapy because she felt "too tired and not strong enough to deal with that."

Through the health maintenance organization, the consultant was also made aware of the fact that 6 months before seeking psychiatric help Mrs. C had attended her family doctor's office on frequent occasions with complaints of fatigue, poor concentration, and weight gain. Aware of her marital problems, the family practitioner had diagnosed depression and prescribed a low dose of amitriptyline, which had made her even more tired and increased her weight further. When she continued to complain and not improve, he had referred her to the mental health clinic.

DSM-III-R

The DSM-III-R multiaxial diagnosis is as follows:

Axis I	Depressive dysthymia (300.40), rule out major depression with melancholic features
Axis II	Personality disorder with avoidant and dependent features (301.90)
Axis III	Rule out hypothyroidism
Axis IV	Severity of Psychosocial Stressors: 3, marital problem, impending emancipation of children, social isolation (moderate–enduring)
Axis V	Current GAF score: 60; highest GAF score past year: 70

Biopsychosocial Matrix

The biopsychosocial matrix is as follows:

	Influences (explanatory—descriptive)	**Interventions (treatment—prognosis)**
BIO	Hypothyroidism Hypothalamic dysfunction (melancholia)	Thyroid panel and thyroid replacement therapy Antidepressant medication
PSYCHO	Susceptibility to loss Critical self-image Desire to excel as a parent Codependency issues	Psychotherapy (including cognitive restructuring) Referral to Al Anon
SOCIAL	Impending emancipation of children Marital issues Absence of extrafamilial reinforcers	Couples therapy Encouragement of increased social life

Biopsychosocial Formulation

This 43-year-old married woman has several developmental issues that render her vulnerable to loss. Her father died when Mrs. C was at an age when she had developed her oedipal attachment but was unable to process the loss. The fact that her mother was forced to work and delegated her care to older siblings was a further symbolic abandonment. While the siblings took good care of material needs, there was a lack of nurturance and a strong emphasis on duty and responsibility, with harsh criticism for failure. This constellation of early events laid the groundwork for adult behaviors that foster depression. Mrs. C is susceptible to loss and withdrawal of affection but subordinates her own emotional needs to the care and pleasing of others. She is determined to excel as a mother in ways that she lacked for herself but is critical of her own performance and has a negative self-image. Most of her energy is expended on her role as mother and spouse, where she has also enabled her husband's alcoholism but is now bitter that he prefers the company of his drinking friends. Other than her attendance at church, Mrs. C has no interests outside the home.

This combination of predisposing social and psychological influences is sufficient to account for Mrs. C's recurrent periods of depression, which are consistent with a diagnosis of dysthymic disorder. These have usually remitted spontaneously when circumstances have changed or when she has mobilized support from her minister. Even between episodes of obvious depression, there are behaviors consistent with a diagnosis of a personality disorder with avoidant and dependent features.

The outside consultant that reviewed the case was struck by the fact that the most recent episode of depression appeared different. It was more severe, and review of both the family practitioner's and the psychotherapist's records suggested that Mrs. C might now be suffering from a major depression with melancholic features. While the impending emancipation of her youngest child could be a sufficient added cause for this, the consultant also noted the atypical feature of increasing weight accompanied by extreme lethargy and wondered if hypothyroidism might be a contributory factor.

It was clear in retrospect that the fact that Mrs. C was referred to the mental health clinic directly by her family doctor led the clinic to waive a psychiatric evaluation. The history of failure to benefit from low-dose antidepressant medication also reinforced the psychiatric social worker's natural tendency to dwell predominantly on social factors and the patient's marriage and to overlook any possible biological contribution.

The consultant recommended that a psychiatrist become directly involved in the care of the patient. A thyroid panel confirmed hypothyroidism. If Mrs. C remained depressed despite thyroid replacement therapy, she probably would respond rapidly to adequate doses of an antidepressant. In view of her weight gain, fluoxetine might be preferred. Once Mrs. C had begun to recover her energy and enthusiasm, she might well accept and benefit from couples therapy, including the possibility of referral to Al Anon to help deal with her husband's alcoholism and her own tendency to enable his drinking. Psychotherapy might also include aspects of cognitive restructuring as well as encouragement to expand her social horizons.

Reference

American Psychiatric Association: Diagnostic and Statistical Manual of Mental Disorders, 3rd Edition, Revised. Washington, DC, American Psychiatric Association, 1987

Index